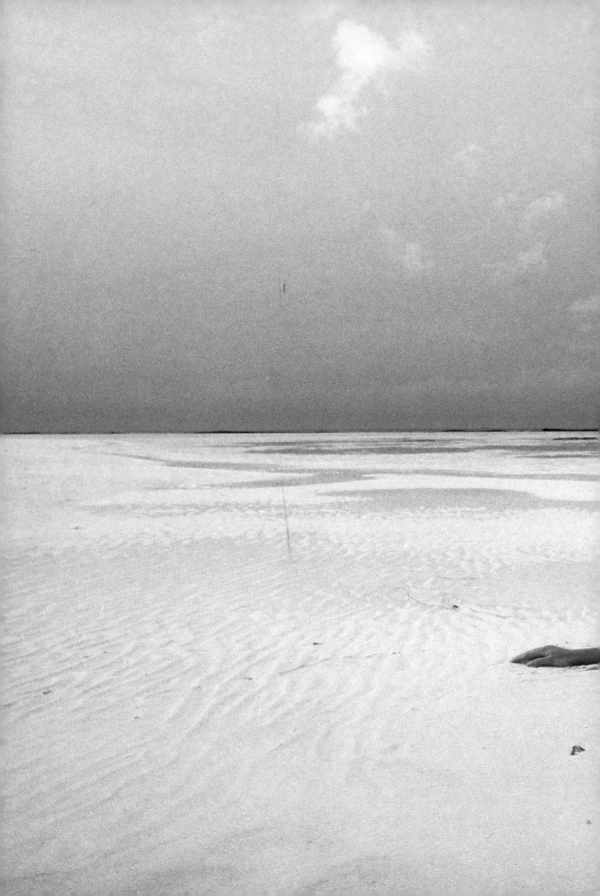

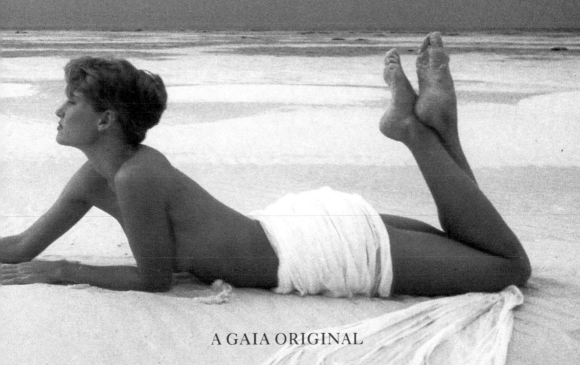

THE BODY/MIND PURIFICATION PROGRAM

By Dr Leon Chaitow

Dr Judy Myers
Consulting Editor

A GAIA ORIGINAL

A Fireside Book
Published by Simon & Schuster Inc.
New York   London   Toronto
Sydney   Tokyo   Singapore

A GAIA ORIGINAL

Written by Leon Chaitow with Angelina Di Fazio (Addictions, emotions and lifestyles p.18-20; and Attitudes, emotions and addiction, p.98-99) and Judy Myers.

DR DI FAZIO has worked for many years as a psychotherapist, specializing in the developmental psychology of women, and in addictions and eating disorders. A former university lecturer and director of clinical services in psychiatric hospitals, she is a sought-after speaker for professional organisations and throughout the business community. She has published widely in Europe, the US and the UK.

Consulting editor DR JUDY MYERS has more than 20 years of experience instituting fitness and wellness programs for hospitals, corporations, health clubs, and alcohol and drug treatment centers (such as Anon Anew and ASAP). She is the coauthor of *Staying Sober: A Nutrition and Exercise Program for the Recovering Alcoholic* and is working on another book about addictions to money, sex, food, drugs, nicotine, and work.

Editorial	Libby Hoseason
	Eve Webster
Development	Rosanne Hooper
	Sara Matthews
Design	Sarah Menon
Illustration	Ann Chasseaud
Direction	Joss Pearson
	Patrick Nugent
Production	Susan Walby

Fireside
Simon & Schuster Building
Rockefeller Center
1230 Avenue of the Americas
New York, New York 10020

First published in Great Britain in 1990
by Unwin Hyman

Printed and bound in Spain by Artes Graficas Toledo
SA D.L. To: 194–1990

10 9 8 7 6 5 4 3 2 1

Library of Congress Catalog Card Number: 90-32258
ISBN: 0-671-68526-0

The information in this book is not intended to replace the services of a trained health professional. Consult your physician or health care professional before following the author's advice or proposed courses of treatment. Any application of the treatment set forth in this book is at the reader's sole discretion and risk.

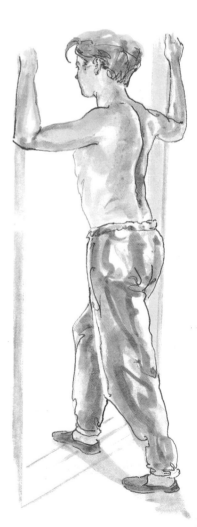

How to use this book

The book is arranged in three major parts —

PART ONE – AWARENESS

This part helps you to identify the scale of the problem —
what state the environment is in, and how your health is
affected by this.

  The Questionnaires on p.43-54 are the key to discovering
how toxic you are. They are described fully on p.43. Answer
them carefully and completely. Follow the advice contained
within them, and then move on to —

PART TWO – DETOXIFICATION

Here are the four programmes which, whether followed
simultaneously or consecutively as appropriate, will take
you from present levels to enhanced health and wellbeing.
Turn to p.56 to learn where to start.

PART THREE – MAINTENANCE

Is self-descriptive. Now the groundwork has been done, this
section is about keeping you well.

  Unfortunately there are no short-cuts. You really do have
to work Parts One and Two to benefit from Part Three —
though you do not have to finish them before you read it.

  To save repetition, there are cross references in the text
where you should look for further relevant information.
Many of the topics covered in Part Three will already have
been raised earlier, and in this case it is intended that you
should refer back.

Conversion table

Imperial	Metric equivalents	
	Approx	Exact
1 ounce	28 grams	28.349
2	57	56.699
3	85	85.048
4	113	113.398
5	142	141.745
6	170	170.097
7	198	198.445
8	227	226.796
16 = 1 lb	450	453.584
2 lb	910	907.168
3 lb	1350	1360.752
0.5 pint		.284 litre
1		.568
2		1.136

Foreword

"All substances are poisons."

This startling statement was made back in the fifteenth century by Paracelsus, the father of toxicology. He went on to say also, "The difference between a poison and a remedy is the dose", a statement based on the fact that toxicity consists of the unbalancing of an organism.

It is the biological accumulation of harmful concentrations of potentially poisonous substances which causes pollution of the environment at large and toxicity in our own bodies.

Thanks to our new-found understanding of the ways in which mind and body can respond to detoxification and health enhancement, we have the opportunity to take responsibility both for ourselves and for our alarmingly polluted world.

Ecological awareness is now evident worldwide. Human ingenuity is as capable of resurrecting and renewing our embattled planet through technology and industry as it has been of assaulting it.

This global "green" revolution can be mirrored by the personal ecological renewal which detoxification of body and mind encourages.

For this there is one primary demand: the acceptance by each one of us of personal responsibility for health and wellbeing. Once this is coupled with the practical employment of safe and effective methods and actions, allied to the marvellous self-repairing mechanisms which operate in all of us, there is no obstacle to the renewal of wellbeing and vigour.

Clear body, clear mind is the objective and, just as the renewal of the planet calls for acceptance of responsibility by all of us, so our own personal "green revolution" calls for determined action and long-term plans.

These are presented in this book.

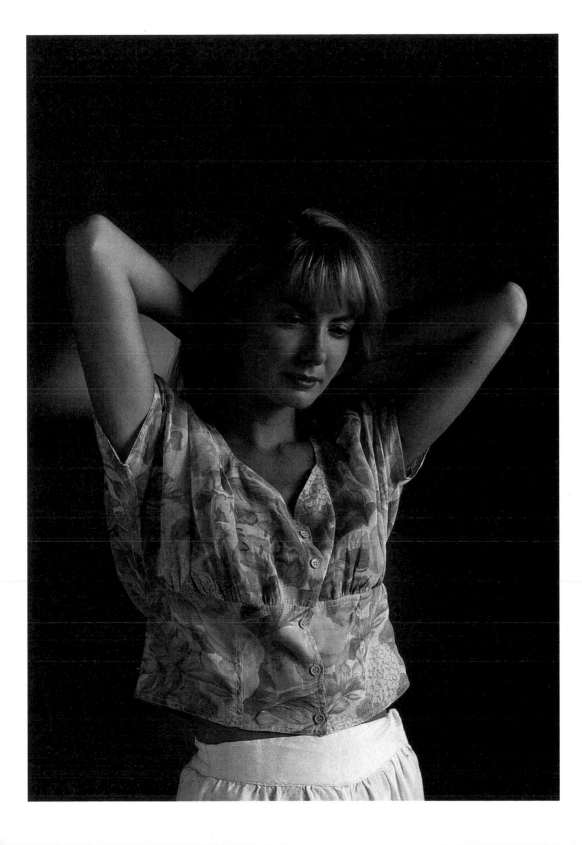

Contents

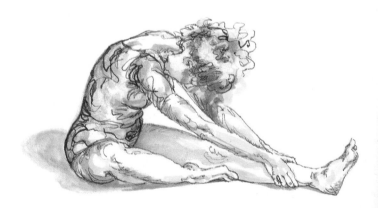

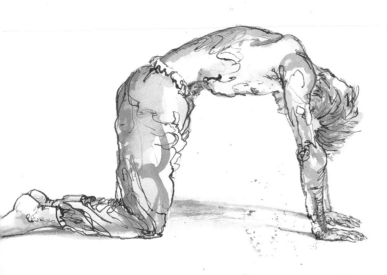

Introduction

Imagine waking in the morning, after about seven hours' deep, undisturbed sleep, feeling refreshed and full of energy. Your bowel movement is normal and regular, your morning meal (as with all the day's meals) is eagerly anticipated and enjoyed. Your day's work, whatever form it takes, is a pleasure not a burden, with only that natural degree of tiredness which results from the concentrated effort you put into all your activities, including those periods of stretching, relaxation and aerobic exercise which punctuate your working day.

Imagine: no headaches, aches or pains, indigestion, skin blemishes, feelings of depression or edginess, or any of the common or "normal" symptoms which seem to afflict most of modern day humans . . . indeed, in this fantasy, you are functioning as you were designed to function, flawlessly, and not, in the words of renowned nutritional scientist, Professor Jeffrey Bland, as one of the "vertically ill", who are not sick enough to lie down, but who are certainly not well.

Compare this image of boundless energy and health with reality, and note the areas where you do not, as of now, meet this ideal. Ask yourself, "Why?". Much may have to do with the way your body is coping with the stresses imposed upon it by internal and external toxicity.

Suddenly the "green" revolution is upon us and every pundit is expounding on the planet's danger from pollution, and the urgency of acting to preserve the fragile ecosystems on which our existence depends. Yet this external environmental pollution is but a macrocosm of what is happening to our own inner ecosystems, to ourselves, to the vehicles in which we exist – our bodies.

Of course we need to pay attention to the outer world, to support and insist upon care of our planet. But is it not also vital that we act to preserve the health and well-being of the body which allows us to perform the multiple activities of a complex and demanding life?

Detoxification of mind and body is part of everyday life. Avoiding contact with obvious toxins, reforming some of the ways you live your life, encouraging active periodic detoxification and focusing on the needs of both mind and body, are strategies to bring that image of boundless energy closer to you.

Do you recall how you felt when you were younger, or how you can still feel after a few days on holiday? Do you remember a sense of wellness which was far more than the mere absence of symptoms? Turning this fantasy back into reality is the aim of the detoxification programme, and it is a goal worth aiming for since full expression of the joy of living is the prize.

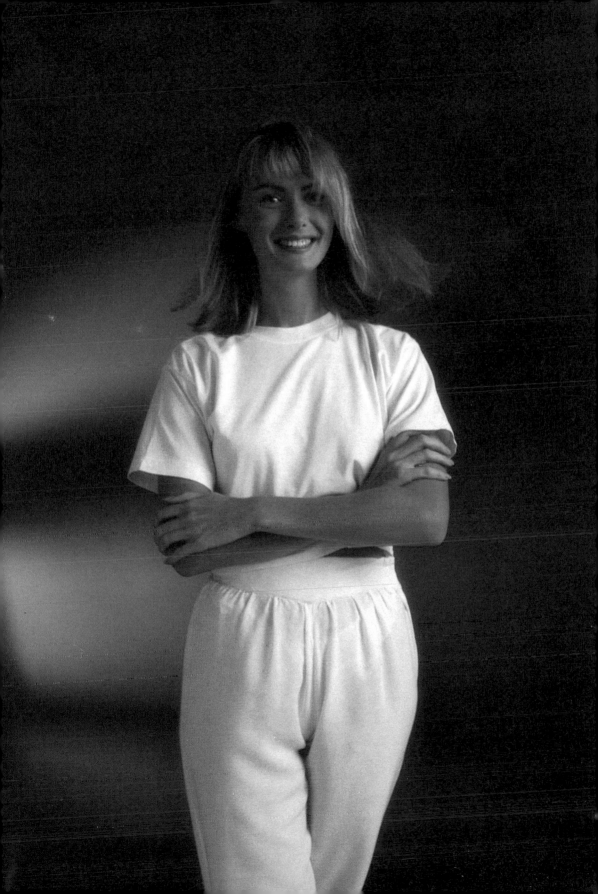

The need to detox

Even engines need periodic servicing and maintenance. The miracle of the human body is that, if we maintain it adequately, to a very large extent it services itself. It is not all that difficult to ease oneself into a pattern in which this maintenance – sound food, adequate exercise and rest, mental and spiritual harmony – becomes the norm. It is also possible, without excessive effort, to give the self-regulating, detoxifying and repairing aspects of the body the chance to become more active.

If we fail to provide our body/mind with such opportunities, a gradual, perhaps almost imperceptible, change takes place, when the efficiency of the self-repair systems goes into decline and greater and ever greater efforts are required to kick them back into action.

It is not normal to feel seedy, low in energy; to be constipated or to have indigestion after most meals; to have skin blemishes and fragile hair; to have lost something of the sense of taste and smell, and to be operating constantly with energy whipped up by stimulants such as tea, coffee, cigarettes or alcohol. If you long to regain that extraordinary level of wellbeing which flows so effortlessly in most children, and which you once enjoyed, then it is time to implement aspects of the programme which follows.

This will call for regular and routine detoxification, using any of a number of equally effective methods, all of which will be explained and described, and which provide a major key to sound health and abundant energy. The initial stages of a detox programme are the most irksome. As you progress, so it becomes easier; and as the levels of toxicity reduce, so the benefits of enhanced health and wellbeing become more established. It is then that the ideal of a well-maintained body/mind complex can be seen to be functioning, with all the gifts of concentration, energy and joy which are our birthright.

Where to start

Your journey of detoxification and repair will be as long or as short as it needs to be. The efficiency of the appropriate organs differs in each one of us, and we all carry differing levels of toxicity, according to what we were born with and what we have picked up along the way. One of the first tasks of the book, therefore, is to identify just where you should start on the programme.

This is done by means of the questionnaires on p.43-54

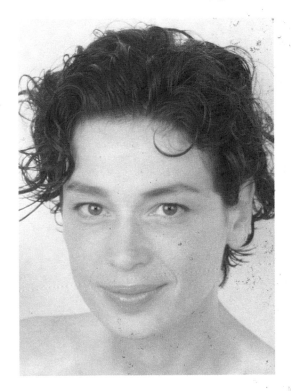

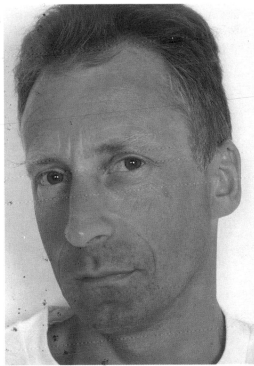

which you are asked to complete carefully. The results will guide you to the various setting-out points.

The many interacting components of a detoxification programme are then introduced to you in appropriate stages, from basic to advanced: various forms of exercise (stretching, relaxation and aerobic) as well as nutritional guidelines and methods for mental stress reduction. A host of methods and substances are included to help make the detoxification process comfortable and safe for you.

Who is it for?

With some exceptions (see below), this programme can be adapted for use by anyone at almost any level of health. Some people, those with diabetes, for example, should take care with some aspects of the programme; wherever there is need for such caution, a note in the text recommends appropriate medical advice should be sought. It is ideal preconception preparation for anyone planning a family.

Certainly anyone living or working in an environment which is polluted should take special note of the many ways available of increasing the defences of the body against pollutants as well as of hastening their exit from the body.

Toxicity has been with us from the very beginning of time, although it is now at the peak of its effect on humans and the planet as a whole. We can choose to defend and protect ourselves, or just blithely ignore what is happening.

For those who choose to confront the challenge this book offers a variety of weapons.

Who it is not for

There may be some people for whom the methods of detoxification may, in principle, be contraindicated. Usually people recovering from active alcoholism or drug addiction, and those people already being cared for by health professionals for the treatment of eating disorders, will find the book both useful and supportive.

It is suggested that professional guidance be sought by anyone concerned about these problems before embarking on any regime which could place the body or mind under further stress. Some addresses will be found on p.187.

PART ONE

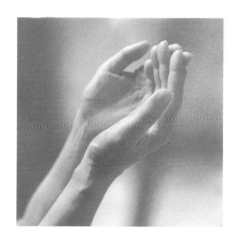

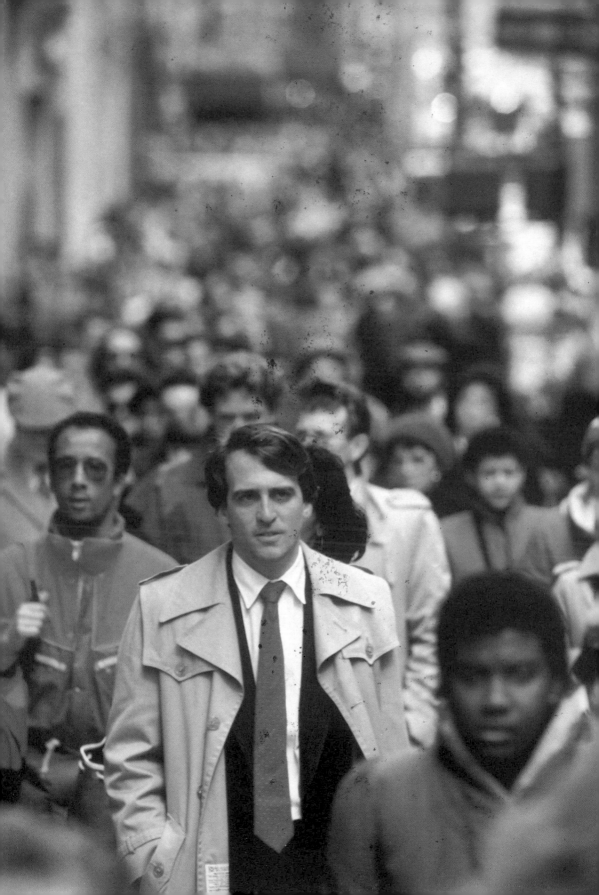

Our toxic society

What do we mean by toxicity? Toxicity may be described as a certain level of all those elements in the physical environment that may be harmful, injurious, unhealthy or, possibly, even lethal. This can include what we eat and breathe, as well as our work and home environment, and we can also include in this definition unhealthy aspects of relationships, destructive social habits, and the toxic effect of living an unbalanced lifestyle.

You may at first be dismayed at the apparently overwhelming array of ways of becoming poisoned, and find it easier to give up before you even begin. Don't be discouraged, though: you don't have to detoxify everything all at once. Take it one step at a time. The purpose of this chapter is to help identify the more immediate hazards so you can make a beginning. It takes time to change the deep-seated habits of a lifetime.

Why do we have to bother at all? Most people look healthy enough and many of us live longer these days. Why not just sit back and enjoy the wonders of modern science? Well, science has provided us with an avalanche of four million new chemical compounds in the past decade, many of them toxic. And many of them combine to create even more poisonous substances, and all too often they end up in our rivers and seas, food chain, drinking water and, ultimately, us.

We are both passive and active recipients of pollutants, poisons, stress, emotional disharmony and many other aspects. Accepting that you will inevitably continue to be a passive receiver of some of them, need not discourage you from getting involved in removing other elements you CAN do something about. You don't have to place yourself at risk in obvious ways – by smoking cigarettes, drinking excessively, eating adulterated foods. Nor do you have to accept debilitating stress, morbific relationships, and destructive thinking and behaviour patterns. And while environmental and atmospheric pollution or radiation may seem to be beyond your control and influence, you can, in reality, take a variety of evasive and protective measures which greatly cut down your exposure and the risk of damage.

Controlling the deluge of toxicity involves making choices. There is much you can improve through diet, lifestyle and behavioural change to cut down toxic input and to reduce harmful levels already stored in your body. This book will show you how to clear out toxins already in your system and how to avoid adding to them. It will also help you assess the less obvious, but potentially even more poisonous, aspects that lie in your attitudes or habitual ways of thinking.

Having profoundly poisoned our planet, we will find it impossible to remove all sources of malign substances from it. As individuals, however, we can regain power of choice over many areas of our lives, through working on the assessments and exercises which follow. This book does not suggest any "quick fix" remedies; that could be hazardous also. But it does recommend that you begin to make changes in your life strategies, based on an understanding of the effects of your current practices on your health.

Addictions, emotions and lifestyles

What creates the strain of modern life? The drive to succeed, fear of failure, breakdown of the extended family, lack of direction, insecurity, emotional stresses, lack of spirituality, social isolation? These are only a few of the dynamics, and all of them bring pressure to bear on you. If you are experiencing feelings of helplessness, inadequacy, lack of self-esteem, or use chemicals or maladaptive coping patterns to deal with these feelings, then your life is overwhelming you and you need to regain control.

People use chemicals, substances or behaviours to change their mood or feelings. The relationship between addiction and feelings is well documented: the only question remaining is which comes first – addiction damaging feelings or difficult feelings causing addiction. But once established, the combination of feelings and addiction dominates lifestyle. A person who is addicted to food, drugs or alcohol will develop a lifestyle which will both protect and support use of the substance or behaviour of choice. Addiction takes a great deal of time and energy.

There are many levels of addiction, beginning with habits, pleasures and stimulants which you think of as "impossible" to give up, as well as those cravings and pleasures you would rather not talk about and which you would probably lie about if asked. These are the things upon which you may become dependent, and may be addicted to. Harmful substances which you cannot stop consuming, using or doing (and stay stopped) without suffering some form of physical or mental discomfort, is something on which you have become dependent. Any substance that you use which regularly dulls, distorts, alters or confuses reality, which stops "what is" from being understood and dealt with, and which you won't give up, is a form of addiction. This is the basis of self-generated toxicity.

Stimulants boost energy by producing adrenalin to allow sugar to be released into the bloodstream. This "upper" triggers insulin release from the pancreas to control your sugar level, thus pushing it down again into a trough where, unable to resist, you take another upper and repeat the cycle, but at increasingly frequent intervals or in greater quantities for the same result. This lift can be obtained quite naturally without flogging your body into exhaustion.

The body produces its own pleasure enhancing and pain killing hormones called endorphins (endogenous morphines) which have similar chemical structures to drugs such as morphine. If you stimulate the pleasure centre in the brain

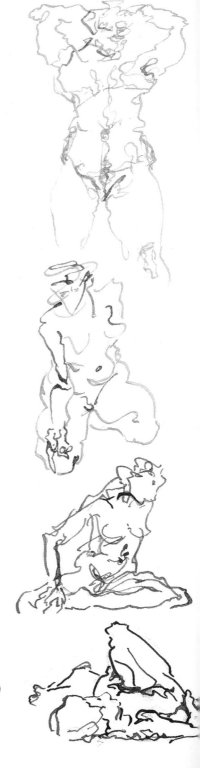

with coffee, tea, chocolate or cola, you use up the natural sources of endorphins. The long-term effect is increasingly destructive, in that it becomes almost impossible to live without such stimulants. Once the natural endorphins have been depleted, people report feeling like "the living dead"; they are awake but no longer have positive or pleasant feelings. It may take months for the brain to restock its supply of endorphins and for the person to begin to feel "alive" again.

Another reason it becomes "impossible" to live without drugs is the intense craving which may be experienced, not only physically, but emotionally, socially and, even, on a cellular level, because the body has adapted to a substance which now seems normal. Once the substance is withdrawn, the body responds on a cellular level by emitting stressors to indicate that it is now out of balance. "Normal" has come to include the once foreign substance, be it alcohol, sugar, caffeine or any other drug.

Most people use substances or behaviours to cope with difficulties, crises or pain at some time in their lives. This may include tobacco smoking, coffee drinking, resort to alcohol or drugs, and inappropriate use of prescriptive medications. In addition, literally millions of people have serious problems with food, either through self-starvation, or becoming entrapped in gorge-vomit cycles. There are also compulsive behaviours such as gambling, sexual permissiveness, or the submersion of self-will in a relationship or religious affiliation.

What is the difference between "use" and addiction? The difference is that non-addicted people stop using when the crisis passes, but the addicted person develops a lifestyle around using, and ultimately loses control of everything.

● Emotions

Emotions are feelings driven by thoughts and actions; they represent the consequence of how you think and what you do. If you indulge in toxic behaviours or substances, your natural emotions will become distorted or lost, leading to two-fold stress: chemical stress on your body and emotional stress on the mind. Because what you think and feel, and how you live are all inextricably linked, the stress build-up will be enormous. It will only be a matter of time before something breaks up under the accumulation of multiple stresses. Will it be your physical health, or your mind, or will your life simply "fall apart"? What is this thing called stress?

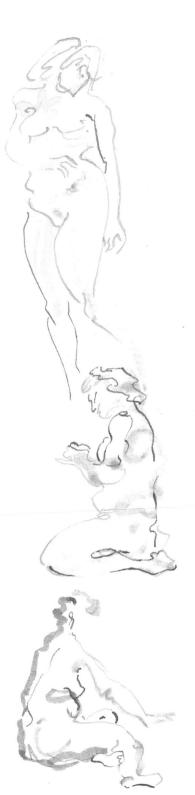

Stress is any demand on your body or mind to respond, adapt, or alter. It is a state of readiness to do battle in order to survive, which requires hyper-vigilance from body and mind. Some stress is necessary to live normally, and, utilized efficiently, can be the opportunity for growth and development, but excessive stress can kill.

More important than the stress level itself is how efficiently you convert it into useful energy. If stress is managing you, rather than vice versa, it can cause destructive change and ill health. Pressures, expectations and demands to succeed, deal with problems, try harder, conform, achieve may all produce enormous stress. It is your emotional reaction that makes the difference between positive utilization and destructive breakdown, especially if many of these pressures or stresses may seem outside your control.

How can you go about breaking the vicious cycle of addiction, stressed emotions, and maladaptive lifestyle – the most toxic combination imaginable – to create a more balanced, natural way of being? You can begin by using the questionnaires on p.43-54 to identify the various factors in your life which need to be changed. When you see how many toxic elements you are allowing into your body and emotions, you may well want to make changes.

Indeed, you can begin to change a little every day. The most profound changes are better made in gentle ways so the adjustment will be easier. It isn't necessary to be hard on yourself, or feel guilty for eating chocolate, or drinking too much wine, or being too dependent in relationships. But it is necessary to do something about it. When you have identified the major areas in which you have allowed toxicity to contaminate your life you can begin making a plan for slow change. A one year plan with monthly and weekly goals will be helpful.

In some instances, you may need professional guidance to solve lifestyle, stress or addiction problems. Some addresses are given in the appendices at the end of the book, which will point you in the right direction.

Personality types (see p. 45)
Type A is: impatient, restless, quick moving, easily angered, not methodical, forceful, competitive, ambitious, punctual, in need of recognition, tense, works to deadlines, unable to relax . . .

Type B is: patient, unrushed, slow to anger, methodical, easy going, not competitive at work or play, happy with present position at work and socially, casual about time, relaxed . . .

Guess who suffers from stress?

How should we respond to our polluted and stressful world? Try to lessen the exposure we receive, and strengthen our own response and hardiness (p. 100).

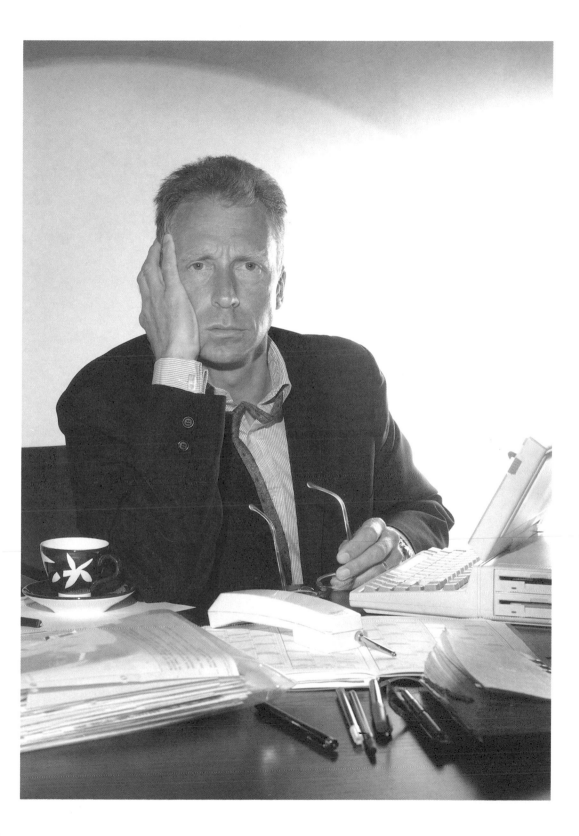

Our sick planet

Our survival depends on the good health of the planet. But the harsh reality is that the planet is sick and getting sicker. Its illness, slow in coming, now involves every facet of the environment which sustains us:

* The ozone layer is under bombardment. Lying in the upper atmosphere 10 to 30 miles above our heads, it protects all life from destructive ultraviolet radiation, a major cause of human skin cancer and cataracts. In some places large holes have opened where up to 50 percent has already been destroyed by gases, especially the chlorofluorocarbons (CFCs) used in aerosols, air conditioning plants, refrigeration and fast food packaging. Each chlorine molecule from CFC can destroy 100,000 ozone molecules in a violent chain reaction.
* The earth's temperature is rising. Gases from human activities, especially the carbon dioxide formed when we burn forests and fuel (wood, gas, oil and coal), trap the heat radiating off the surface of the earth. Methane from farming, nitrous oxide, and water vapour also trap heat, as do CFCs. Each molecule of CFC traps 20,000 times as much heat as one of carbon dioxide. This "greenhouse" effect will result in the gradual melting of the ice caps and cause ocean levels to rise. Meanwhile radical changes in climate and weather will be here within a few decades.
* Poisons now rain from the sky. Acid rain can destroy trees and the creatures living in lakes and rivers, leaving them sterile and lifeless. Even virgin polar snow and ice can now be polluted and acidic.
* Millions of tons of human and industrial waste are poured into our waterways every year, gradually poisoning our rivers, lakes and oceans. When the dry summer of 1989 lowered water levels in the River Ouse, the villages round Drax power station in south Yorkshire were sprinkled with sewage particles drawn up into the atmosphere by its cooling system.
* Tropical forests are being ripped out and burned, depriving the earth of its climate-moderating green cover, and irreplaceable resources, while species vanish forever and atmospheric pollution increases.
* Agricultural soil now often contains pesticide and other chemical residues; poisons from the soil enter into the water passing through it, and the crops growing on it, and so into us. Your health, which depends on the quality of your food, ultimately depends on the quality of the soil.

Does this really matter to you? Consider:
* Serious allergic disease (immune system damage) among children in the UK has increased six times over the past 40 years.
* All human breast milk, whether in the jungles of South America or urban Los Angeles, is now contaminated with traces of dioxin and other toxic environmental chemicals.
* You now have around 100 times more lead in you than did your grandmother's grandmother.
Yes, it matters.

The air we breathe   Mood changes, allergy, visual and mental disturbance, rashes, flu-like symptoms, nervous system disorders, and, above all, respiratory disease are some of the consequences of just breathing. Indoors or out, we regularly take in the products of combustion (whether from heating, cooking, vehicle emissions or refuse disposal), which are highly carcinogenic, as well as asbestos, lead, pesticides, petrochemical vapours, formaldehyde, radon, sulphur and nitrogen dioxide and second-hand cigarette smoke.

Sunlight and cancer   Light is the basic life-source on the planet. Unfiltered daylight – not necessarily direct sunlight – is a daily requirement for nourishing the body; people who are deprived of full-spectrum light can become depressed and develop behaviour problems (see p. 118). But sunlight also contains radiating wavelengths, an overdose of which can cause skin cancer and the production of free radicals (see p. 36). The best protection is an intact ozone layer; clothing, sunscreen lotions containing the B vitamin PABA, and the antioxidant vitamins A, C, and E all help.

Radiation   All species on earth have evolved to thrive at an ambient level of background radiation – whether from cosmic sources or the Earth itself. However, high local doses of radioactivity are carcinogenic. The largest single source of these is radon – a naturally occurring gas in certain rocks, especially granite, also found in some building materials, such as concrete, bricks and tiles. If you suspect you live in a radon area, seek professional advice from your local authority or ecological group. Preventive measures are available.

Water   Tap water can now be one of the most regular sources of toxicity to which we are exposed. Drinking water derived from wells is very often contaminated, by wastes, pesticides and other toxins. Furthermore, unless the water is very hard, it can leach and carry with it heavy metals from either copper or lead pipes; these can lead to mental retardation in children and to nervous system illnesses. Chlorination to control bacteria is also a hazard: a recent National Cancer Institute survey showed that in ten areas of the US, regular consumption of chlorinated tap water was responsible for between 12 and 27 percent of bladder cancers. The only safe water is pure spring or filtered water.

Common ingredients of tap water are: petrochemical derivatives,(benzene, carbon tetrachloride), heavy metals (mercury), dioxin, agent orange, DDT, polychlorinated biphenyls, asbestos, arsenic, vinyl chloride, chlorine, pesticides, nitrates and nitrites from fertilizer . . . and many more. Many are carcinogens or cause birth defects.

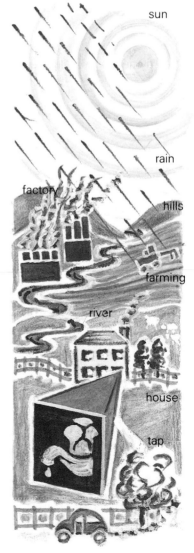

sun

rain

factory

hills

farming

river

house

tap

Food and farming

Pesticides, insecticides and herbicides kill the rodents, insects, moulds and weeds which interfere with economic crop production. However, they do not vanish after doing their job, but linger in our food, soil, water — and us.

The dangers of these substances have been known for years, but the extent of the danger is now such that economic considerations will have to give way to health as pests become more resistant and chemicals more deadly.

Tolerance levels are alarmingly low: eating more than a mere 7.5 ounces of aubergine (egg plant) a year exposes you to an unsafe level of *legal* pesticide residue, according to US Environmental Protection Agency figures.

Meat, poultry and milk production tell their own horror stories. Poultry, constantly dosed with antibiotics for their own limited survival, pass on ever more disease-resistant bacteria. The result is that at least 35 percent of all factory farmed chickens sold in Britain, Europe and America are contaminated with salmonella. Many farm animals are over-confined and dosed with antibiotics to keep disease down, dosed with hormones for more rapid growth and eventually slaughtered in ways which cause rupturing of the intestines and contamination by faeces.

Milk from cows intensively fed and medicated like this carries drug residues and contaminants; food-poisoning bacteria can survive normal pasteurization. Seventeen thousand people were poisoned by contaminated milk in the mid-West states in 1985. Further outbreaks of listeriosis (30 percent are fatal) in pasteurized milk took place in Mass., in pasteurized cheese in Ca. (1987), and in Britain in 1989.

* Alternative biological methods of pest control are being developed: harmless (to crops and us) parasitic insects can kill plant pests; sterile female pests can interfere with reproductive cycles; more refined application of current pesticides can take the place of blanket spraying; and organic (non-chemical) food production is developing.
* Take precautions: wash all hard-skinned produce in well-diluted washing- up liquid (rinse well). Remove the outer leaves of leafy vegetables, peel waxy coating off fruit and vegetables, and try to grow your own or buy organic produce where available.
* Buy organically cultivated meat and lower your intake of dairy products. Regular supplementation with friendly bacteria (high potency acidophilus) and the eating of live yogurt, will reduce your chances of succumbing to attack from salmonella and listeria.

In 1940 only seven species of mites and insects were resistant to chemicals; the figure is now 450.

The US National Academy of Sciences estimates one million cases of cancer over the next decade from pesticides in food alone (i.e. excluding other pesticide risk from water and atmospheric contamination). Forty percent of domestic and 60-70 percent of imported food in the US now contains measurable pesticide residues. Ironically, pesticides banned in the US or UK may be manufactured for export to the Third World, and contaminated products then come home to roost.

Out-of-season fruits and vegetables carry double the risk of pesticide and fungicide contamination — and 90 percent of fungicides are carcinogenic.

The chemical fertilizers used in intensive farming destroy the microecology of the soil. More chemicals are then needed to produce the same crop. Crops in enfeebled soil become less resistant to disease, so ever more biocides are required; the toxic spiral continues, with literally unquantifiable consequences as chemicals build up in the food chain. And fertilizer residues, some of them potential carcinogens (nitrites) also get into the water chain, contaminating rivers, lakes, oceans, and us.

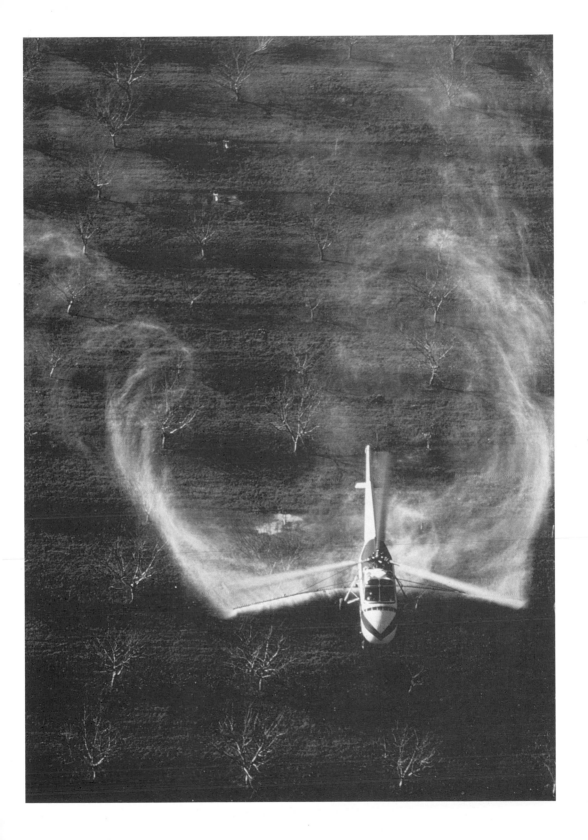

Food processing

A degree of processing is necessary to make much of the nourishment of food available to us. For example, heat breaks down cellular fibres to release essential vitamins and other nutrients. Too much heat, however, and those same nutrients are destroyed. This balance, between benefit and damage, is especially critical in the use of preservatives and additives.

Traditional methods of preserving food include salting, smoking, adding sugar, drying, pickling , chilling, or a combination of these. To these are now added refining, freezing, canning, chemical treatment and irradiation. All damage the food to some extent (see p. 128-9), but some are more safe than others.

Additives   are used to increase shelf-life, retard spoilage, simplify preparation, enhance flavour and sweeten. Some are essential if our present range of foods is to remain available, but many are harmful, especially to sensitive individuals who may suffer violent allergic reactions, and others are highly toxic. Legislation governs permitted additives in most countries, and regulates appropriate labelling.

Irradiation   replaces dangerous substances such as sodium nitrite in prolonging shelf-life, and killing insects. parasites and bacteria; it is claimed to inhibit the sprouting of vegetables and ripening of fruits. Objections to its use are grounded on the free radical activity (see p. 36) it generates, the chemical compounds it may create in food and its destruction of vitamin E. While its use is sanctioned in the US for pork, spices, fruits, vegetables (with poultry and fish probably coming soon), some European countries, including the UK, have not yet allowed it.

Freezing   is one of the best means of preservation; disadvantages are limited to some loss of nutrient value and textural quality. But look out for added sugar in, for instance, peas and colouring additives. **Sun-drying** is also a good method, though sun-dried foods, especially fruits, have a high fungus (mould) content. **Chemical drying**, is now the commonest method, and the sulphates used are undesirable in any quantity. **Pre-cooking** leaves critical safety factors in manufacturers' hands. If meat and dairy stuffs are not cooked for long enough at the correct temperature, contamination by such bacteria as salmonella and listeria may remain to survive inadequate storage and rewarming in the home, canteen or restaurant.

Experts continue to debate the safety of some additives such as aspartame, used as a sugar replacement in 'diet' drinks and foods. It is 200 times sweeter than white sugar.

Its predecessors, such as cyclamate, were withdrawn as possible carcinogens. Although given a clean bill of health by authorities, high intakes of aspartame have been linked to neurological and other symptoms which have reversed when intake has stopped.

When aspartame is digested, it breaks down into methanol, better known as wood alcohol. After your enzymes have digested this, it may end up in your bloodstream as formaldehyde, the chemical used to preserve dead bodies, with unpredictable toxic effects.

Our modern diet

There is just too much evidence to doubt the positive correlation both between diet and health, and between diet and behaviour.

Increased life expectancy figures conceal the fact that although more of us reach age 40 due to lower infant mortality and fewer deaths from infection, the quality of life is declining and survivors to this age do not now, on average, live longer than they would have 40 years ago. Moreover, serious diseases such as cardiovascular degeneration, high blood pressure, arthritis and cancer are starting sooner, often in childhood. Much of this can be traced to deficient diet.

In adults the effects are also clear. Despite increasingly available medical care, chronic illnesses (cardiovascular disease, cancers of all sorts, neurological diseases and arthritis) are on the increase. Surveys in the US (Jersey City) showed that 88 percent of adults have a deficiency of one or more essential nutrients in their bloodstreams; 64 percent were deficient in two or more vitamins. Similar studies in Europe show much the same picture. When we add such deficiency to known toxic factors we have a deadly combination. The result: average length of life the same; health quality drastically down. Not quite what we had hoped for.

Allergy is a very common result of inappropriate diet, and allergic reaction plus toxicity can be a dangerous combination. Toxins entering the body by whatever route have to be dealt with by the immune system and the organs of detoxification – the liver, kidneys and skin. If allergy already exists, they will already be under great strain. With more exposure to irritating toxins, your whole body may become sensitized and produce increasingly violent allergic reactions. This commonly happens with certain foods, especially those introduced to your diet in early infancy if there was little or no breast feeding. This is why wheat, eggs and, above all, dairy produce, are the commonest allergens.

If such foods are introduced gradually or eaten frequently, the allergic reaction, if any, may become "masked", i.e. there is no single violent reaction, but many minor ones; these can cause a host of physical and mental symptoms. An important alarm signal that masked allergy is present is the development of a craving for that food. Special rotation diets (p. 136) can help to overcome this.

The World Health Organisation estimates that more than three quarters of all cancers are diet related. This is now thought to hold true for other chronic diseases.

The British Society for Population Studies said in 1985 that children are now six times more likely to suffer from eczema, and three times more likely to develop asthma than in 1945.

Studies in the US show that if the diet of delinquent children is changed to no-milk (a common cause of allergy) and low-sugar, their behaviour improves dramatically. When dietary and chelation methods (p. 117) are used to remove heavy metal contamination (such as lead, mercury, cadmium) a similar improvement is also seen.

Toxicity at home and work

Despite their slick decor, many modern offices are seething with noxious toxins which may account for your feeling dizzy, headachey, fatigued or just plain out of sorts, and for smarting eyes and breathing difficulties. Over 20 percent of employees in a quarter of all modern office buildings suffer *acute* discomfort while at work.

The fault usually lies in poor design, allowing a combination of unsatisfactory movement of air, hazardous fumes, excessive temperature, low levels of negative ionisation and lack of humidity. Of pollution, the US Environmental Protection Agency says that the air in some offices is a hundred times more polluted than the air outside.

Air conditioning, and heating and ventilation systems are a marvellous breeding ground for undesirable (even lethal) fungi, moulds and bacteria, especially if they are regularly turned off at night or weekends. These organisms are then liberally distributed throughout the building when the machines are switched on again.

Shops are risk areas too: we find particularly high toxic levels in copy shops, office equipment suppliers, dry cleaners (carbon tetrachloride is especially toxic), hair dressing salons, electrical supply and repair shops, motor repair shops, furniture, carpet and interior decor suppliers (foam in furniture, synthetic materials), and paint and decorating materials suppliers.

Most office pollution comes from sources such as copying machine chemicals, carbonless paper, paint, rugs, curtains, wall panelling and cleaning solvents, most of which exude such vapours as formaldehyde, a chemical which is capable of causing skin rashes, nausea and menstrual irregularities. It is one of the most powerful sources of free radical activity (see p. 36); its influence is more obvious in new buildings than old.

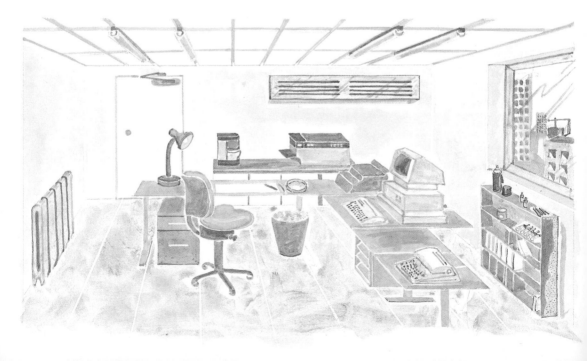

Your home may also be full of hazards – even from seemingly innocent sources. The fabric of the building itself (walls, floors, insulation), timber and dampproofing treatments, paints, chipboards, plastic tiles – all these contribute their share. Always be on guard for reactions caused by the products you use, question the need for some of the aids you are accustomed to, and demand and get non-toxic substitutes wherever possible. Here are some common horrors:

* dish or clothes washing: calcium sodium edetate or phosphate compounds can penetrate the skin; they are toxic irritants.
* paper towels: formaldehyde is a paper-strengthening agent (skin rashes, nausea, menstrual irregularities). Bleached paper contains dioxin.
* air freshener: carbolic acid or formaldehyde. And check for CFCs.
* cleaning the oven: the main ingredient of most cleaners is lye, one of the nastiest toxic substances around. Phenols, formaldehyde (again), benzene or ammonia can bring blisters and rashes to the cleaning of baths or similar surfaces.
* furniture and tile polish: sodium phosphate or turpentine may penetrate the skin or get inhaled as vapour.
* toilets: cresol, a major germ-killer, is easily absorbed through the skin and can damage major organs. Deodorant blocks depend for "effectiveness" on your breathing their vapours. Scented paper is more irritant than plain; white may have been chlorine-bleached.
* drains: lye, again, or sulphuric acid. Avoid contact with either, or expect major skin problems.
* clothes: benzene, sulphamic acid or toluene for spot removing cause skin rashes and, perhaps, complications involving the nervous system. Shoes : nitro-benzene turns skin blue, affects breathing and induces vomiting.
* swimming? Wash yourself thoroughly after immersion in chlorinated water. Gardening? Satisfy yourself about the consequences of *any* spray or fertilizer before touching it. Cooking? Remember the dangers of inhaling fumes and steam; some vapours from deep frying oils may be carcinogenic. Use your ventilator and stand back.

It would be absurd, even if possible, to isolate oneself completely against these hazards. However, non-toxic alternatives do exist. Where they don't, take simple precautions, wear protective clothing, and, when in doubt, leave it out.

Toiletries

Use cornflour or arrowroot instead of talc; bicarbonate of soda instead of antiperspirant (aluminium chlorohydrate blocks pores); regular washing plus essential oils instead of the strong chemicals in deodorant.

Your teeth do not need the ammonia, ethanol, formaldehyde, mineral oil, saccharin, sugar or PVP plastic ingredients of commercial pastes; use bicarb and peppermint oil, or natural herb pastes available from health shops.

Your scalp needs regular brushing and massage not toxic anti-dandruff shampoos. Good general health will be more effective than these in remedying this condition.

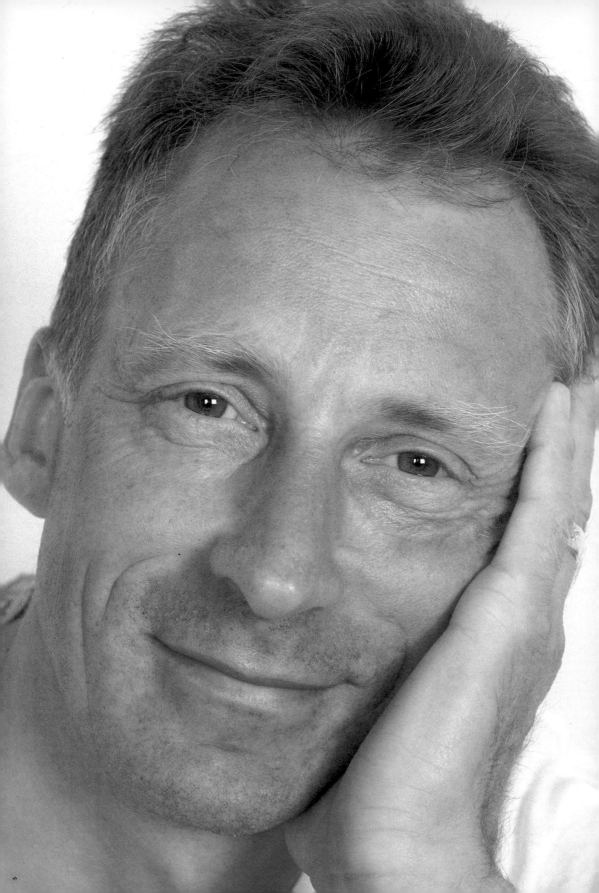

The bodymind fights back

Your body does not passively soak up toxins like a sponge. It has defences and resources which act constantly, even while you sleep. When toxins enter your body they can be swiftly dealt with, provided there is an efficient response. The younger and healthier you are, the more appropriate that response is likely to be and the less damage your body will suffer. The older, or less healthy, the poorer the protective response and the greater the likelihood of damage to your body.

The elimination of toxins by your body is not just a matter of getting rid of poisons which arrive uninvited in food, drink or air, or through contact with your skin. It is a non-stop campaign to get rid of the toxic debris left over from the very act of living.

This complex process of detoxification involves the immune system (especially the white blood cells), the lungs, kidneys, bowels, liver and the skin. Overseeing and coordinating all of this is the mind.

The process of energy generation, in which raw materials such as fats, proteins and sugars are broken down and used to energize the body, leaves wastes behind just as ash and clinker are left in a furnace. This is one of the major sources of toxic waste in your body.

All body cells have a finite life and are constantly being replaced. Some of their useful amino acids and essential fatty acids can be reused; other products are of no further use and are added to the refuse awaiting disposal. The job of reprocessing self-generated toxic materials and recycling useful materials is done by the liver and various enzyme systems. Other debris is eliminated in urine and faeces, by exhalation (an amazing amount of junk leaves your body via the lungs) or through the skin.

Your multi-faceted immune system can take care of irritant substances present in food, drink and the environment. For example, when your eyes smart in a smoky room or smog-laden city street, damage is being done to you by free radicals (see p. 36). By becoming watery-eyed, however, your system delivers soothing anti-oxidant substances to neutralize the irritant toxins. Some other toxins, such as those associated with alcohol, are not so easily dealt with and require that major organs of detoxification, such as the liver, operate on them to render them harmless. The liver may eventually become overwhelmed by the volume of toxins foisted upon it.

The bowel is an important area for efficient detoxification. If local conditions are abnormal, due to poor dietary habits, constipation or other reasons, putrifying food residues may become toxic and enter the bloodstream, slowly poisoning you. At this point other less obvious organs of elimination such as the skin may then come into operation to try to put matters right.

Through all this, the state of your mind is critical to your body's efficient detoxification activity. A basic understanding of how the body works, what helps it and what harms it, is a huge step foward in the direction of health. Attention to diet, exercise, emotional harmony, tidying up lifestyle habits, and a range of simple but effective methods which help detoxification, can improve all aspects of this self-cleansing process.

The toxin fighters

Cut yourself or break a bone and, usually, your tissues will heal without any direction from you. Equally, your kidneys, liver and other major organs work with no conscious effort on your part. These are some of the self- healing, self-regulating, self-balancing functions of your body in action, known as homoeostasis. It is homoeostasis which keeps you alive and on which you rely to detoxify your body every moment of the day and night.

The efficiency of your homoeostatic functions depends on what you have inherited, and what you have acquired, along the way. Some people seem to get away with almost anything they do to their bodies (see box), while others can cope with very little toxic or emotional stress. There is, as we will see, a lot you can do about improving your own levels of homoeostasis.

Stress factors challenge your body or mind to adapt or alter in three stages. The first is the alarm stage when there is a quick alteration of body processes, such as a rise in heart rate and blood pressure, perhaps to cope with an emotional demand. If that demand is repeated frequently, the body stops reacting quickly, and goes into the adaptation stage. Now the heart rate and blood pressure, say, would be permanently raised, and stay that way until the body was no longer able to sustain this effort. The final stage, collapse, appears, perhaps after many years, in which adaptation fails and illness or death results. All this applies to toxicity as well.

As undesirable substances come into contact with your body, inside or out, there is a reaction against them. Smokers may remember this from their first cigarette. If the irritant is repeated, the body adapts and reacts less violently as it becomes "sensitized" to the substance. Eventually you will learn to live with the poison through heroic efforts on the part of your organs of elimination and detoxification. In time dependence or actual addiction may develop, until eventually the powers of adaptation – detoxification – can no longer cope, and collapse takes place, with disease or death the inevitable result.

What decides how well you cope with toxicity and stress? Your health is the result of your inherited genetic make-up and all that you have done to yourself and had done to you up to this time. It is this level of susceptibility, the efficiency of your homoeostatic functions, and the power of the toxins you are exposed to, which decide how much harm will come to you.

Tough cells
Cells taken from various tissues of elderly but healthy life-long smokers were compared with cells from bronchitic life-long smokers. It was found that the cells of the healthy smokers were "tough": they could be exposed to almost any highly toxic substance without being easily damaged. The reasons for this are not understood, but it explains why some people get away with the way they treat themselves. Most of us, however, need to work at achieving protection.

The immune system

Everyone in the age of AIDS has heard of it, but if you were asked where your immune system was, what would you say? In your bloodstream? Your nervous system? Hormonal system? Digestive system? The spleen or liver? Your mind? Well, it is in all of these, and everywhere else in your body as well.

Your immune function involves cooperative operations by different mechanisms and cells. It constantly watches over every aspect of the defence of your body, especially against toxicity. There are many ways of improving its function when it is poor, and some surprisingly common substances can also depress it when it is healthy. Here are some of the nutrients which can do this.

Nutrient:	Boosts	Depresses
Sugar		Macrophage activity
Selenium	Primary response	
Extra Vit C	Overall resistance	
Vit C deficiency		Inflammatory response
48 hour water fast	Cell mediated immunity	
48 hour plus fast		Cell mediated immunity
Iron deficiency		Host resistance
Excess iron		Host resistance
Excess polyunsaturated fatty acids	T & B cell function	Proliferation response
Excess or deficient zinc		Cellular immunity

Liver   This cleansing, manufacturing and storage centre performs over 1500 different functions. It processes all foods (except for some fats) absorbed from the intestines before they are released into the bloodstream. It also filters the blood, removing, deactivating or reprocessing wastes, toxins and bacteria. It deals with everything, even alcohol and pesticides, but overeating and excessive exposure to toxins of any sort, will overload the liver and weaken its ability to detoxify. Through its influence on nutrient and energy supply, as well as detoxification, the liver has a direct link with the mind and its function.

Lungs   The lungs help clear the system of toxic debris; it is carried away by the enormous amount of water vapour exhaled daily – far more than you pass as urine. Bad breath is often entirely due to bowel putrefaction, though other causes are also possible.

Inhaled pollutants reach the bloodstream more rapidly than those arriving in food, as there is less filtration protection in the lungs. Carbon monoxide and nicotine from tobacco smoke are the single most important causes of lifestyle death today, from cardiovascular disease and a variety of cancers.

We can use our lungs to poison ourselves or to detoxify our system, as well as to calm the nervous system and induce relaxation (see p.63).

Skin   The skin has a remarkable detoxification function. If the body cannot use its normal routes of elimination efficiently, the skin will be used instead, and blemishes, pimples, boils or rashes may be a consequence. Elimination through the skin is an important part of a detoxification programme (see p.159).

Kidneys   The kidneys not only take toxins from the blood for elimination in the urine, they also salvage and reabsorb valuable nutrients, which are then recycled for further use in the body.

These wonderful filters gradually decline in efficiency as you get older and excessive toxicity due to diet, drugs or environment will place strain on them; and liver problems, too, cause them overwork. Any weakening of kidney function affects the heart, and vice versa.

Lymphatics   A vast network of vessels carry lymph around your body. This is part of an intricate waste disposal and nutrient supply system, which interacts with the blood-stream through special ducts. Lymphatic motion, however, depends mainly on the pumping action of breathing, and of muscles as they contract during use. All lymph passes through the filtration of a lymph node before leaving a vital organ. Nodes are also the sites of manufacture or storage of major immune function agents such as the lymphocytes and macrophages, cells which protect against infection, cancer, and toxicity. You may recognize such nodes in your neck; they swell when you have a throat infection or cold.

Intestines and the friendly bacteria.   As food passes from the stomach into the intestines, its nutrients are absorbed, and its residue left for elimination. Hundreds of billions of microorganisms are involved in this process; without them you could not survive for long.

Inside your intestines live about 400 different species of uninvited residents, weighing between them 3–5 pounds

(1.4–2.3 kilos). Some, such as the friendly bacteria Bifidobacteria and Lactobacillus acidophilus, are truly amazing
agents of detoxification. They help digest your food, stimulate normal peristaltic action (the movement which pushes
bowel contents along) and control some of the less desirable residents of your bowel, such as Candida albicans (see
p. 38), as well as actively cancer-causing chemicals.

This happens because what suits you also suits them: the
ammonia, cholesterol and carcinogenic toxins which would
damage you are meat and drink to them, and in acting first
to kill disease-carrying bacteria, they are acting in self-
defence. If we live on a diet which contains a lot of fat and
sugar, and excessive red meat, however, we stop them
from functioning normally, and lose most of their benefits.
We also damage them by using drugs such as antibiotics
excessively. These do not differentiate between disease-
causing and friendly bacteria, and kill both. If on the other
hand we feed them a diet which is rich in complex carbohydrates (vegetables, fruits, nuts, beans, and whole grains)
they thrive and so do we.

Recent research has shown that the friendly bacteria of
breast-fed babies have changed over the past 40 years.
They used to be more resistant to infection than bottle
(formula) fed babies. Between 1950 and 1989 a change has
taken place in mothers' milk. Worldwide, Bifidobacteria
fragilis is in decline because of pollution; all breast milk now
contains pesticides and other toxic residues which damage
these microorganisms.

Fortunately we can supplement infants with this bacterial
culture, and also supplement ourselves if our microecology
has been damaged by poor diet or medication. Just how
important a healthy bowel ecology is, is seen in the so-called
gay or toxic bowel syndrome. A combination of drug and
dietary abuse as well as repetitive sexually transmitted
infections destroyed the bowel health of many people, who
later went on to develop AIDS and other immune-dificiency
related diseases.

If we want good health and detoxification, we have to pay
particular attention to this most vital region, and to its
remarkable, anonymous inhabitants.

Toxic overload

In good health the liver, lungs, skin, kidneys, lymphatics and the rest of the immune function deal with toxins as they arrive in the body. Unfortunately, if for any reason these detoxification processes weaken and adapt (see p. 32), toxins will be allowed to accumulate and symptoms such as allergies, fatigue and skin problems will appear.

A deficiency of specific nutrients, for instance, may allow some toxins to produce severe damage to our cells by a process called free radical oxidation (see below). Oxidation also occurs dramatically quickly when fats, inadequately protected by antioxidants such as vitamins C and E, become rancid. Too much cholesterol/fat present in your arteries causes oxidation, damage to their lining and, eventually, arteriosclerosis.

Oxidizing heavy metals such as lead, excessive iron or copper, and cadmium produces similar damage; as do the free radicals in smoke and alcohol. Cells so affected can become cancerous or part of an arthritic or any other inflammatory process.

You can protect yourself by avoiding accumulations of free radical generating substances – toxins, fats, metals and smoke – and by a diet and supplements which supply antioxidant substances such as vitamins A, C, and E, minerals such as selenium and zinc, and amino acids such as cysteine (found in garlic).

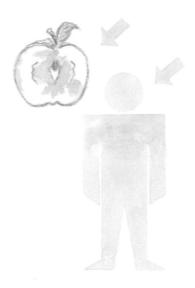

Free radicals
A free radical is a rogue molecule with a free attachment arm, hell-bent on grabbing part of another molecule with that arm. It usually chooses an electron from a normal molecule, which itself becomes damaged and unstable and with a free arm of its own.

We can see this destructive chain reaction happening around us in metal as it rusts, rubber as it perishes, and apples and potatoes as their cut surfaces turn brown. Similar processes also take place inside us, rapidly when tissues are in contact with toxic substances such as strong acids (see p. 28-9), or more slowly when fatty substances in our bloodstream oxidise (become rancid) or as we age. For it is largely free radical activity which causes our cells to age and protein synthesizing machinery to become less efficient. It is this that causes skin to wrinkle, and muscle tissue to harden with age.

Signs and symptoms of toxicity

Some consequences of toxic damage are obvious: diarrhoea consequent upon food poisoning; severe lung irritation from exposure to pungent fumes; severe burning by contact with bleach. Toxic exposure, while less acute, may not be so easily recognised. Be suspicious of strange signs and symptoms without obvious cause: those that occur at regular intervals; those that persist such as skin rashes; unexpected fatigue or muscle aches, headaches, metallic taste, digestive problems (nausea, cramp, diarrhoea, bloating), frequent upper respiratory irritation (mucus accumulation, sneezing, recurrent "colds", persistent cough), itchy or red eyes, and all-too-frequent mood changes, including depression, anxiety, hyperactivity or inability to concentrate, and extreme sleepiness.

These same symptoms are also found in allergic conditions, but since allergy is a uniquely abnormal response, you are likely to be the only one affected; as toxicity is a universal response you may expect others to become ill as well as yourself.

Heavy metal toxicity is a common air and water pollutant; symptoms should always set alarm bells ringing. Lead, aluminium and cadmium produce headaches, hyperactivity, behavioural changes, memory lapses and learning disabilities. Mercury causes nervous system symptoms (numbness, tremors, loose teeth and bleeding gums, paralysis, poor coordination). Hair analysis is a simple way of discovering whether heavy metals are currently poisoning you.

Try to find causes rather than just relieve the symptoms. For example, it is better to avoid eating foods containing monosodium glutamate than kill the pain of the headache it causes. Understand that diarrhoea is a serious attempt by the body to get rid of what is not wanted, so don't just take medicine to overrule the body's homoeostatic effort. Find the cause, take plenty of liquid and rest until the body has done its clearance job.

Using a cortisone cream to clear a skin rash will prevent you from discovering that it is caused by your newest soap. Hyperactive children who are given tranquilizers may develop long-term dependency or addiction. A real cure is only possible if the toxic or allergic cause of their behaviour is discovered. Short-term use of anti-depressant drugs is helpful only for severe depression. Find the toxic, allergic or emotional cause and deal with that; the depression will lift.

Travellers tips
For two weeks before travel to anywhere food and customs are different or hygiene unreliable, take a quarter teaspoonful of high potency acidophilus powder (one that requires refrigeration) in pure water, twice daily, away from meals. Continue this throughout your stay, increasing to hourly doses if diarrhoea occurs (in which case also call a doctor and drink plenty of bottled or filtered water). For two weeks before and throughout the stay, also take a gram daily of vitamin C to enhance immune function.

Candida

Yeasts such as Candida albicans live in our intestines. They do no harm unless the balance of bacteria which control them is weakened. One of the major controls is a B vitamin, biotin, manufactured by healthy, friendly bacteria. If they are damaged, and biotin manufacture ceases, a dramatic altera-tion takes place in the yeast: it spreads and changes into an aggressive fungal form, putting down root-like structures which penetrate the lining of the bowel and allow absorption into the bloodstream of partially digested food fragments, yeast breakdown products and other toxic substances, which provoke allergic and immune system reactions.

The exact sequence of Candida spread varies: other health prob-lems already in existence, and in-born differences determine the exact progression. If left untreated, this rampant activity can affect every aspect of life and health, mind and body. Widespread candidiasis is the first alarm signal in the onset of AIDS. Many believe it even predis-poses the immune system to this ultimate collapse.

The yeast can spread to other parts of the body, causing inflammation (thrush) and a host of other symptoms (see below). The activity of the fungus causes progressive dam-age to the immune system.

Those most prone to Candida overgrowth are people who have had hormone treatment (including long-term use of the "pill"), more than one pregnancy, several short or one long course of antibiotics, exposure to toxic substances, or who have a high sugar/fat intake.

The yeast can be controlled by supplementation with high potency friendly bacteria, a low sugar diet, no yeasts in the diet, and specific anti-fungal medications, including biotin, olive oil and garlic.

Something happens
(see text above)
and then:

Yeast spreads
and becomes fungal

Digestive symptoms
(bloating, diarrhoea, heart-
burn, constipation), sugar
craving, general tiredness

Acne and other skin problems
(athlete's foot, fungal nail changes)

Allergies, menstrual problems, PMS,
cystitis, vaginitis, thrush (oral or vaginal)

Anxiety, depression, mood changes, irritability,
migraines, extreme tiredness, sleep disturbance,
loss of concentration, loss of libido, sense of hopelessness

Severe immune suppression, chronic fatigue syndrome, extreme
susceptibility to infection, multiple allergies (food, substance, environment)

Emotional symptoms with chemical causes

Agoraphobia and hyperventilation Fear of open spaces locks people into a prison of their own making. It is the result of anxiety and is often accompanied by acute panic attacks. This may be triggered by hyperventilation – a habit of overbreathing which changes the blood chemistry and nervous system behaviour within seconds.

Heavy metal and chemical toxicity are sometimes the starting point for phobic behaviour and panic attacks, but a more common cause is excessive sugar intake which often ends with a state of chronic hypoglycaemia (low blood sugar). Its symptoms are anxiety and panic attacks and a tendency to fainting. You only need pass out once on a bus or in a shop to feel the first protective need not to go outside again; the phobia or "unnatural fear" has begun.

Cycles of high and low blood sugar are produced by substances such as coffee, tea, alcohol, cigarettes and cola drinks. First they stimulate adrenalin production which forces sugar release into the blood; then the body pushes this down again with insulin.

Depression and hyperactivity Neurotransmitters are the key to your changes of emotion. They increase or decrease the transmission of messages to and from the brain. When those which improve transmission are in excess, behaviour is hyperactive (manic); an excess of those which slow transmission down brings lethargy, indifference and, probably, depression.

Deficiency in essential nutrients, the presence of toxic substances and a variety of drugs including cocaine, marijuana, steroids (the "pill" causes major nutrient imbalances), and the beta-blockers used for treating high blood pressure and heart disease, all influence neurotransmitter function. So, too, do heavy metals such as mercury, lead and cadmium, all high in depressed people; but the more common causes are the daily tasty toxins found in coffee, tea and cola drinks.

A recently identified cause of depression is excessive use of aspartame, the artificial sweetener now widely used in diet colas. It is made up of amino acids which, when metabolized, cause an imbalance in brain chemistry because of their extreme concentration.

Studies have shown a direct link between the degree and severity of psychiatric illnesses such as depression, and the amount of caffeine consumed. Caffeine has a direct effect on brain chemistry as well as an influence on sugar levels.

The immune system is directly controlled by the mind. The science of psycho-neuro-immunology has clearly established that negative emotions and thought patterns (hate, fear, anger and jealousy) reduce the efficiency of the body's defences.

We can poison ourselves by thought just as efficiently as by chemicals, and detoxification means we need to pay attention to both these possible sources of toxicity.

Psycho-neuro-immunology: the mind/body link

In 1975 Dr Robert Ader was conditioning rats to dislike sweetened water by injecting them with a chemical to make them feel ill whenever they drank it. After the injections had been stopped for some time, some of the rats began dying and, on investigation, Ader found that the chemical he had used was a suppressor of immune function. The rats had not only become conditioned to feeling ill whenever they drank sweet water, they were also mimicking its other effects and depressing their immune systems. This ability to depress their immune function was proof positive of the nervous system's control over the immune system. Many tests since then have confirmed this in humans.

A study at Oxford University's Common Cold Unit showed that some people with stressful life experiences during the previous six months had more severe colds than did others with the same stresses. The difference? Those worst affected had introverted personalities and found it difficult to become involved in life (see the hardiness factor on p.100). Poor stress-coping skills and negative emotions are immune-suppressing and predispose to infection and ill-health. If there is also nutritional deficiency and exposure to toxic materials, there is double vulnerability.

The important lesson to be derived from this is not that some people become ill when faced with stress and negative emotions, but that many people facing the same stresses remain healthy. We can learn to copy and apply positive emotions and coping skills, as a means to prevent illness, to cope with it when it exists and to accelerate recovery from it.

Positive emotional counselling and methods of mind control, including visualization and guided imagery techniques (see p.110) have proved helpful for people with even such serious illnesses as cancer and AIDS. If such methods can prove effective there, they can certainly be used for less serious health problems.

One of the pioneers of psycho-neuro-immunology, Dr George Solomon, says a "distress-free" state of mind is needed for a strong immune function. This requires happiness, a sense of control, relaxation and positive emotions.

A healthy immune system protects you not only from infection and toxic substances, but also against cancer. If immune surveillance is poor, cells which are becoming cancerous may not be spotted and dealt with efficiently. Woody Allen once said, "I don't get depressed, I grow a tumor instead." Many a true word is spoken in jest.

Natural Killer Cells and emotions
Students are known to be more prone to infection before exams. A vital part of defence against infection comes from Natural Killer Cells (NKC), the activity of which is itself easily studied. It was found that students who scored high in psychological tests showing them to cope poorly with stress had weak NKC activity at exam time (and when they were lonely); these were the students who became ill. The journal reporting this (The Lancet, 27 June 1987) states "It is the individual's response to stress that determines the effect on immunity, not the stress itself".

Positive action

We have now seen some of the ways in which we can be exposed to toxic materials and emotions. Equally, we have also seen something of our resources, the homoeostatic mechanisms by which our organs of elimination and our powerful immune system protect us against, deactivate, and eliminate toxins of all sorts.

When you have completed the series of self-assessment questions on p.44-54, the programmes which follow will show you how to apply elimination strategies to get rid of those toxins presently in your body. They also explain more fully the long term strategies for avoiding toxicity and actively detoxifying that have so far only been touched on.

You will be asked to pay close attention to what you eat and drink. This is fundamental to detoxification and, if attended to, will give you a higher level of wellbeing than you have known before.

What is good health? It is certainly far more than just an absence of illhealth. Our aim is vital health, an energetic and positively exciting state of body and mind which allows for a creative and fulfilling life. This calls for some effort, but it is worth it. You will be taking charge, and accepting a large measure of responsibility. The rewards will be correspondingly great.

As well as the dietary changes and choices which will be spelt out, you will be asked to take action in the areas of lifestyle and exercise. As with the dietary programme, this will be tailored to your particular needs based on the answers you give on the next few pages.

You may be asked to begin with the Modified detoxification programme because of particular health problems, or because of the volume of toxicity or stress which you are currently coping with. You will also be asked to follow a sequence from basic breathing exercises through relaxation and on to meditation and visualization. Additionally, a number of specific techniques and methods will be presented to you so you can learn to use the detoxification potential of your body to the full.

After detoxification, the Maintenance plan is provided for long-term health protection and stability. As you detoxify and learn to relax and cope with stress, to use the various forms of detoxification enhancement, as well as the nutritional and exercise strategies, you will sense the dawning of a new era for yourself.

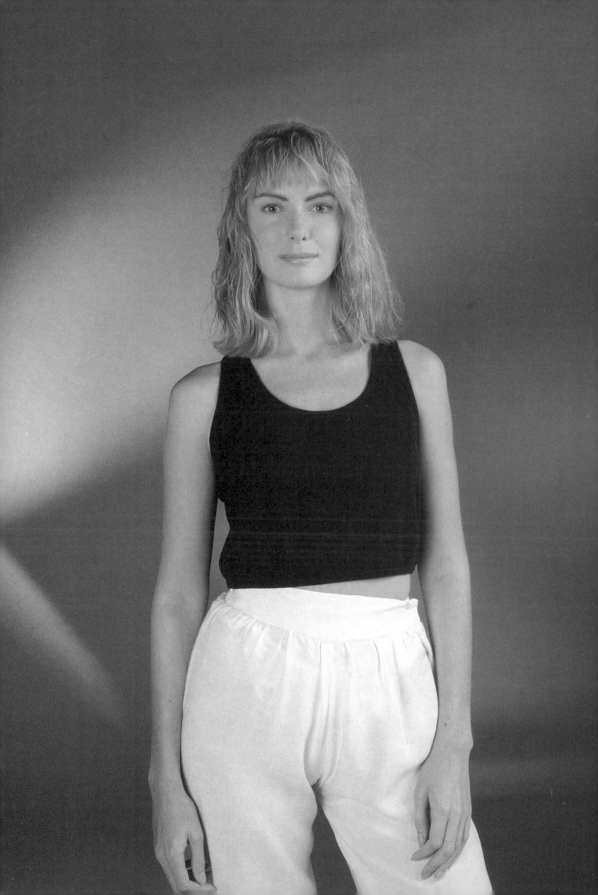

How toxic are you?

The aim is to help you achieve better high-level health and wellbeing through detoxification. A necessary preliminary to a detoxification programme is to draw as detailed a profile of you and your needs as possible. This is done by asking questions about you and your lifestyle.

Most people will benefit from following the programme in different ways because of their different requirements and vulnerabilities, so guidance is needed in identifying problem areas and particular needs.

The questionnaires on the following pages are designed to do just that. They will help you to assess

* your level of health,
* how much stress you face,
* how healthy your diet and lifestyle are,
* the hazards you face and how you cope with them.
* whether you get enough sleep, relaxation and exercise,
* and something about your attitudes to life.

Through some of the questions you may identify certain health problems, such as diabetes or allergy, which require that you seek advice before making changes to your diet, or, such as cardiovascular disease, before starting the exercise programme. Other questions may reveal particular needs such as preliminary emphasis on stress reduction. It is all too easy to ask too much of our marvellous adaptive capacities, especially if we are already coping with toxicity, stress or ill-health.

Each section is a unit, and will give you advice based on your score within that unit, and also on your individual answers, so is tailored to your unique needs. This advice should take precedence over that given on p.56-7. If you are referred to the Maintenance programme, even at an early stage, you should carry on to complete all the questionnaires since there may be other problems that you need to know about. The scores will form a useful record to check how your health has improved as a result of the actions you take.

When you have finished the questionnaires, turn to p.56-7. There you will be directed to the appropriate starting gate on the basis of your cumulative score over all the questions, so it is vital that you answer all the questions.

Answer as honestly and accurately as you can, short of worrying about it. The correct answer is usually the one you first feel like giving as you read the question, not the one you are tempted to give after pondering and agonizing.

In some sections accuracy is bound to be variable. Some answers will be direct YES or NO; in others, though, we have to accept a certain vagueness. Don't worry, just put down what you feel intuitively is your closest assessment of accuracy. Just do your best.

Your willingness to start a detox programme shows your willingness to take responsibility for your health. Do not be dismayed by the difficulties involved in restructuring your life to achieve this. Provided you are satisfied that the answers you have given are accurate to the best of your ability, this book will help you lead a healthier and more fulfilling life.

Lifestyle

Answer the questions in the following four sections HIGH (score 3) if that is true more than once a week, MEDIUM (score 2) if only once a week, and LOW (score 1) for less than once a week.

● **Work patterns**
1 Do you sit or stand for prolonged periods at work?
2 Do you have to lift things, bend, twist, or perform repetitive actions for most of the day?
3 Do you have to use machinery that makes your body, or part of it, vibrate, for long periods?
4 Is your work area noisy, uncomfortable, overcrowded, or poorly lit?
5 Is your work ever physically dangerous or emotionally draining?
6 Do you work near electric or electronic equipment (computer screens, switchboard)?

If you answered YES to questions 1, 2 and 3 pay particular attention to the stretching and aerobic exercises in the programme and apply the methods on p.104-5.
   If you answered YES to questions 4 or 5, concentrate on the relaxation exercises (p.64).
   If you answered YES to question 6, take a daily supplement of 200iu vitamin E to reduce the effects of low-level radiation and read p.122-4 for advice.
   If your total score is more than 12 in this section, work is a major stress source in your life. Attention to relaxation and detoxification can be of great help to you.

● **Time management**
1 Do you do shift work?
2 Do you work more than eight hours every day?
3 Do you often work for more than five consecutive days?
4 Do you ever get less than one hour for your lunch break?

5 Do you get less than two *consecutive* weeks annual holiday?
6 Do you regularly have to work to deadlines?

If you scored more than 8 points in this section, go to p.97-9 for general guidance about stress.

● **Sleep**
1 Do you get less than 7 hours of sleep in 24 hours?
2 Do you have difficulty getting to sleep at night?
3 Do you often wake at night and are then unable to get to sleep again?
4 Do you have very disturbing dreams?
5 Do you use medication or alcohol to get to sleep?

If you have scored more than 6 in this section, then your sleep pattern is probably affecting your ability to function well. The Detox programme will help you, but see also p.100 for more specific advice.

● **Personal space and relationships**
1 Do you feel that you haven't got enough time to deal with everything you have to do?
2 Do you fail to get at least one and a half hours a day to yourself?
3 Do you fail to get enough time (for you) to spend on your hobbies, or worse still, do you not have time for hobbies at all?
4 Do you have too much free time with nothing to do?
5 Are there days when you speak to no one except when shopping or other casual conversation?
6 Are there days when you don't touch anybody, and nobody touches you?
7 Do you feel that you lack companionship?
8 Do you have difficulties over your sexlife?
9 Are you preoccupied with sexual matters?

10 Do you feel unappreciated?
11 Are there personality clashes at home or at work?
12 Do you feel "taken for granted"?
13 Does life seem meaningless and without purpose?
14 Are you living with an alcoholic or addict, or with someone disabled or dependent?
15 Are you a single parent?

If you answered YES to questions 1 to 3, you need to reexamine your priorities and devote more time to yourself.

If the answer to question 4 was YES, consider getting a job or taking an interest in either a creative hobby or voluntary work where you can help others.

If your total score for this section was more than 10, you need to pay particular attention to stress-reducing in both the Basic (p.62) and Maintenance (Part 3) programmes.

● **Exercise and relaxation**

This section helps you assess whether you are doing enough physical exercise and relaxation to reduce stress and preserve your health. Follow the instructions in each question on how to score. The importance of each kind of exercise will become clearer as you progress through the detox programme.

1 How often do you practise some form of relaxation exercise?

If you spend at least a 20-minute period (or two ten-minute periods) daily doing some form of relaxation exercise, such as yoga, meditation, Tai chi or breathing, score 0 and move on. If not, then score according to how often you do some kind of relaxation exercise in every week as follows:
1 – more than twice but not daily
2 – at least twice a week
3 – less than once weekly or never.

2 How often do you do some form of aerobic exercise in every week?

Score 0 if you already do at least 30 minutes of aerobic exercise every other day, or train twice weekly in an active team sport. If not score as follows:
1 – more than twice weekly, but not regularly on alternate days
2 – twice weekly on your own
3 – less than once a week.

3 How often do you do some form of stretching exercise in every week?

Score 0 if you spend at least 15 minutes every other day doing stretching exercises (e.g. yoga) on your own, or if you go twice weekly to a class. If not, score as follows:
1 – more than twice, alone, but not regularly on alternate days
2 – twice, alone, or once weekly, in a class.
3 – once, alone, or less than weekly in a class, or never.

● **Personality Types**

Research has shown that personality and behaviour can influence our chances of developing stress-related illness, such as cardiovascular disease.

Study the lists of traits below, and tick those which are more typical of you to find out if you are Type A or Type B.

○ *Type A characteristics*

Cannot stand delay, very impatient
Walks, moves, eats, and talks quickly
Restless and anxious, if not busy
Easily angered by people, events
Works quickly, not methodical
Often does two things at a time
Forceful, dominant personality
Extremely competitive, must win
Seeks advancement, socially and at work
Craves public and peer recognition
Sets and works to deadlines
Always punctual and time conscious
Facial muscles taut, may have nervous tics
Clenches fists, hands never still

○ *Type B characteristics*
Patient, delay causes no anxiety
Walks, moves, eats, talks without rush
Happy to be idle
Difficult to arouse, slow to anger
Slow steady worker
Does one thing at a time
Retiring, easy-going, not pushy
Not competitive at work or play
Content with present position
No interest in opinions of others
Ignores deadlines
Not time conscious, casual about time
Relaxed facial muscles
Composed, hands relaxed

Score 3 for each Type A indication. Type A personalities are most vulnerable to stress and stress-induced illness. Just three Type A indications can mean that stress is affecting your health. If you have ticked seven or more, you should seriously consider modifying your habits. Try to mimic one Type B aspect at a time, until you become comfortable with it. Relaxation techniques described throughout the book and the methods on p.64 will also help.

● Dependent personalities
Answer the following questions YES or NO. Score 1 for each YES.
  1 Do you feel that other people's opinions and values are more important or accurate than your own?
  2 Do you need someone else's approval or regard to feel "good" about yourself?
  3 Are your main activities centred around satisfying the needs of others or one other person?
  4 Have you put aside your own hobbies and interests to involve yourself in someone else's?
  5 Do your long-term plans revolve around another person, and would you do anything to preserve this relationship?
  6 Does fear of someone else's anger or disapproval determine your actions?
  7 Do you use "giving" (of yourself, effort, things) in order to feel safe in a relationship?
  8 Has your social circle become smaller because you involve yourself with just one person?
  9 Does the quality of your life vary with that of one other person's (or group of people)?
  10 Are your efforts largely focused on making someone do things "your way"?

If more than one of these is YES, you may have a tendency to undervalue yourself, and to seek approval and reassurance. This is not necessarily "bad" but it may be stifling your potential. You would benefit from contact with like-minded people, perhaps in a group setting, in order to realize your abilities.

● Addictive personality
The following questions will help to identify addictive behaviour patterns. Answer YES or NO, and score 3 for every YES. Try to answer these questions with painful honesty, otherwise you may be masking the signs of a serious problem.
  1 Do you feel isolated and afraid of other people, especially those in authority, and feel frightened by anger or criticism directed at you?
  2 Do you judge yourself harshly and have low self-esteem?
  3 Did you answer three or more of the questions on dependency with a YES?
  4 Do you feel responsible for the problems of others?
  5 Do you find it difficult to recognize and express your deepest feelings?
  6 Do you confuse love with pity, and love people whom you can pity and rescue?
  7 Do you get "high" on excitement, danger, argument or crises?
  8 Do you crave a food or substance at least once a week?

9 Does yielding to such a craving make you want more, either immediately or soon afterwards?
10 If you "give up" one substance you crave, do you replace it with another?
11 Have any members of your family had addictions to substances or activities?

If your total score is above 6 for the first six questions and you answer YES for any of questions 7 to 11, then you may have a tendency to addiction which you can do a great deal to overcome. See p.99.

● Stress
Some stress is helpful. Each person has a different positive stress threshold beyond which it becomes destructive. Some people show remarkable abilities to withstand extreme stress; the characteristics which allow them to do so have been termed "the hardiness factor". Interacting coping skills can be learned if they are missing in your makeup. Answer the following questions YES or NO and score 3 for every YES.
1 Do you find it hard to involve yourself actively in what other people are doing around you?
2 Are you disinterested in (and avoid involvement with) other people, social activity, local affairs, team games?
3 Do you feel that "things" happen to you (or your family) which you can neither control nor overcome?
4 Do you see changes as threatening to you and your pattern of life, rather than as challenges?
5 Do you feel that life is meaningless, a series of whims of fate over which you have no control?

If you score 3 or more, try to encourage the development of the hardiness factor in yourself. Read p.100.

Habits

For questions 1, 2, 11 and 14, score 3 for once a week or more; 2 between once a week and twice a month; 1 for less than that but many times a year. YES for any of the other questions scores 3 if this occurred within the past year.

● Alcohol use
These questions refer to alcohol, but also apply to any other substance, or even behaviour, which you may use regularly.
1 Do you use alcohol to unwind or sleep?
2 Do you drink to get yourself going?
3 Have you embarrassed, frightened, or hurt yourself by drinking?
4 Has your work been affected because of drinking?
5 Are you defensive when asked about your use of alcohol?
6 Has your recall of events ever been affected by drinking?
7 Are there times when you have to have a drink?
8 Have you tried to stop or reduce your intake but failed?
9 Do you drink enough to get drunk when you are alone?
10 Do you ever lie about how much you consume?
11 Do you use alcohol medicinally or to alter your mood and abilities?
12 Would you find it difficult to give up drinking for three months?
13 Are you angry with yourself that you can't control your drinking?
14 Do you wake with a hangover?
15 Do you ever feel uncomfortable leaving a drink unfinished?
16 Might you have a drink problem?

Any YES answer shows some symptom of a drinking or drugging problem. If your score is above 7, consult a specialist and read p.97-101.

● Smoking
1 Do you smoke tobacco every day?
2 Do you smoke 20 cigarettes/
   ½oz tobacco/5 cigars a day or more?
3 Do you live or work with smokers?
4 Were you a smoker, but quit less than a
   year ago? (If YES score 2)
5 Did you try to stop, but failed?

If your score is above 3 you need to protect
yourself from the effects of smoking. Consider
getting help in order to break the habit. Read
p.97-101 and p.183.

● Caffeine
Do you eat/drink more than:
1 Two cups of coffee daily?
2 Three cups of tea daily?
3 One cola drink daily?
4 Three chocolate products weekly?
Have you ever:
5 Tried to stop using any of these and
   failed?
6 Used any of them to aid concentration,
   or get a "lift"?

Any YES answers may mean that you are dependent upon these stimulants. Read p.97–101 and
p.183 for advice.

● Prescriptive drugs
1 Have you taken a weight-reducing drug
   for more than three weeks?
2 Have you taken sleeping tablets or tran-
   quillizers for more than two weeks?
3 Have you had any amalgam fillings this
   year and/or have you more than four
   fillings altogether?
4 Are you defensive when questioned on
   your use of prescriptive drugs?
5 Have you taken any form of contracep-
   tive pill for more than a year?
6 Do you take prescription drugs other
   than as advised by your doctor?
7 Have you embarrassed or upset yourself, while using medication?
8 Are you becoming dependent on your
   medication?
9 Do you find excuses to keep taking any
   particular drug?
10 Might you have a drug problem?

If you answered YES to questions 6 to 10, seek
professional advice. If you answered YES to
question 3, see p.117. If your total score is
above 9 read p.97-101 and p.183.

Note: if the total score of the four sections
(alcohol use, smoking, caffeine and prescriptive
drugs) is above 20, go to the Modified Dietary
Detoxification Programme, p.86. See explanation on p.56.

Environment

Answer the questions on this page either YES or NO. Score 3 points for every YES unless a question specifies otherwise.

● Work place toxicity

1 Do you come into contact with, or in close proximity to, toxic chemicals or industrial byproducts, or is your place of work in a smog-laden area, or do you work in a dental surgery?
2 Is your place of work air-conditioned, centrally heated, or double-glazed?
3 Are there electrical or electronic machines operating near you?
4 Is radiation used anywhere near your usual work position?
5 Are there any high-voltage power lines over your place of work?
6 Are you in daily contact with cleaning materials through your work?
7 Have colleagues complained of "sick-building syndrome"?
8 Do you work in any way with poisonous metals or asbestos?

If you answered YES to any of the above you should take half a gram of vitamin C, daily. Refer to p.113-14, 121 and 126 for advice on dealing with toxins. For question 8, you should also read p.117.

● Home toxicity

1 Is your house air-conditioned, centrally-heated and/or double-glazed?
2 Have you had the walls of your house insulated with foam?
3 Do you have synthetic or vinyl-backed furnishings/upholstery in your home?
4 Are your water pipes lead or copper? (Score 2 if they are, but 3 if you are also in a soft water area.)
5 Do you handle normal household cleaners and polishes almost daily?
6 Is there a lot of granite, or underground water sources in your area and/or is your house made largely of stone, cement or concrete?

7 Have you had any kind of interior decoration done in your home within the last six months, or is your home in a smog-laden area?

If any of these are answered YES, take half a gram daily of vitamin C (unless you already do so). Refer to p.113-26.

● Travel

1 Do you fly more than once (return) in each year? (If YES score 1)
2 Do you take transcontinental flights more than once a year? (If YES score 3)
3 Do you travel more than 100 kilometres daily by car, on average? (score 1 if in country area, 3 if in city)
4 Do you travel by public transport in a city four times a week, or more?
5 Are you active outdoors, in a city centre, for more than 30 minutes most days?

If your score is above 3 you are exposing your body to pollutants and oxidants. Read p.28-39, and refer to p.113-26.

● Leisure

1 Do you swim in chlorinated water more than once weekly?
2 Do you exercise on city roads more than twice weekly, for more than 30 minutes at a time?
3 Do you participate in motor sports?
4 Do you paint for a hobby?
5 If DIY is a hobby, do you use sprays, varnishes, paints, glue, sanding or polishing equipment, or inhale wood-dust, brick powder, or other fumes?
6 Do you service and/or maintain your own car as a hobby?
7 Do you use chemical pesticides or ferti-lizer in your garden?

If you answer YES to any of the above you are adding to your toxic burden, even though these activities do some good through relaxation. If questions 5, 6, or 7 were answered YES read p.28-39 and apply the advice on p.113-127.

Diet assessment

As you answer these questions, your personal need for dietary change will become clearer as you identify imbalances, toxicities, and deficiencies. Use the questions to guide you to the changes that you need to make.

The questions can be answered OFTEN (more than twice weekly), score 3; SOMETIMES (less than twice weekly but more than three times a month), score 2, SELDOM (one to three times a month), score 1, or NEVER (less than once a month), score 0. Some questions give individual guidance on how to score.

● Imbalances

1 Do you eat canned vegetables?
2 Is your breakfast just a beverage, such as coffee, or nothing at all?
3 Do you snack on pretzels, crisps, salted/roasted nuts?
4 Do you eat TV dinners or prepared meals requiring only re-heating?
5 Do you eat frozen vegetables?
6 Do you drink diet soda or cola?
7 Do you eat at fast-food restaurants or snack bars?
8 Do you add salt to your food at table?
9 Are there days on which you eat no fresh fruit? (If YES score 3)
10 Are there days on which you eat no raw or fresh vegetables? (If YES score 3)

If your score is above 10, try to modify your eating habits to bring the score down to 5 at most. If it is above 20, you really need to adopt more wholesome eating habits. These will become clearer as we progress with the detox programme.

● Fats and oils

1 Do you eat *any* fried food?
2 Do you eat food fried or roasted in butter or animal fats?
3 Having cooked with oil or fat, do you ever heat and reuse it?
4 Do you eat full-fat cheese (e.g. cheddar) or more than half an ounce of butter or margarine daily?
5 Do you drink full-fat milk or use cream (more than just a touch)?
6 Do you eat the skin of poultry, however it is cooked?
7 Do you eat red meat?
8 Do you eat processed meat products?
9 Do you eat bought biscuits, pastries, cakes or crisps?
10 Do you eat brains, liver, heart, or kidneys?

If your score is above 10, try to bring it down to 6. If the score is above 15, you are endangering your physical health through excessive fat intake; the programme will reduce this to safe levels. The questions themselves should guide you to the changes you could make.

● Protein

1 Do you eat less than, 3 ounces of animal protein or 5 ounces of a combination of cereals and pulses, every day? (If YES, score 3)
2 Do you eat more than 8 ounces of animal protein daily?

If you answered YES to question 1 you are not getting enough protein. Vegetarians must ensure a combination (see p.85).

If you answered YES to question 2, reduce protein intake and supplement your diet with 50mg of vitamin B6 daily.

● Carbohydrates

1 Do you consume more than two teaspoons of sugar, honey, or syrup a day?
2 Do you eat sweets, or chew sugary gum?
3 Do you eat "fruit-flavoured" yoghurt or any ice-cream?
4 Do you eat jams or preserves on bread, toast, or biscuits?

5 Do you use sauces such as tomato ketchup, Worcester sauce, brown sauce?

6 Do you eat white bread, pasta, and rice in preference to "brown"?

7 Do you eat processed cereals in preference to sugarless granola or muesli, or oatmeal for breakfast?

8 Do you have a "sweet" dessert?

9 Do you drink regular colas or sodas?

10 Do you drink fruit juice (either fresh or canned)?

11 Do you eat any dried fruit?

12 Do you eat canned fruit?

If the score is above 12, reduce your sugar intake and take 1g daily of the amino acid L-Glutamine; drink water between meals to reduce sugar craving.

Answer the following sections either YES or NO. Score 3 for a YES and 0 for a NO unless otherwise indicated.

● Toxicities

1 Do you drink more than one and a half glasses of wine, or one pint of beer, or any spirits daily?

2 Do you drink more than one cup of coffee (even decaffeinated) daily?

3 Do you drink more than one cup of tea daily?

4 Do you eat or drink chocolate?

5 Do you drink tap water, or use it for making tea or coffee, or for cooking?

6 Do you eat barbecued foods?

7 Can you ensure that your vegetables are organically grown and free of pesticide sprays? (If NO, score 3)

8 Can you ensure that your meat/poultry/eggs are free-range and that no hormones/antibiotics have been used in their production? (If NO, score 3)

9 Can you ensure that all food you consume is free from added colouring and flavouring? (If NO, score 3)

10 Do you remove all skin from fruit before eating it? (If NO, score 3)

11 Do you discard the outer leaves of leafy vegetables? (If NO, score 3)

12 Do you scrub and peel all non-organic root vegetables? (If NO, score 3)

If the score is above 15, try to reduce it to 8 or less. If the score is above 20 take a supplement of either L-Cysteine or Glutathione.

● Deficiencies
(Possible deficiencies in brackets)

1 Are you losing your hair and is it becoming very fine or breaks easily? (Protein)

2 When you clean your teeth do your gums bleed? Do wounds or cuts heal slowly? (Vitamin C and/or zinc)

3 Is your tongue very red or red at the tip, sore or very sensitive to heat? (Vitamin B-complex)

4 Have you a poor sense of taste or smell? Do your nails have white flecks? (Zinc)

5 Are you pale, easily tired, and are the whites of your eyes slightly blue? (Iron and/or Vitamin C)

6 Do you recall your dreams on waking? (Vitamin B6)

7 Do you get cramps at night? (Calcium and/or magnesium)

8 Do you have trouble seeing in moderate darkness? (Vitamin A)

9 Do you have very rough, dry skin on the elbows or knees? (Vitamin A)

10 Does it take a long time for your cuts to stop bleeding, or do you have frequent nosebleeds? (Vitamin K or C)

All YES answers in this section indicate probable nutrient deficiencies which should improve as the programme of detoxication unfolds. If ANY are answered YES take a good quality multivitamin/mineral tablet daily.

Ailments

● **Diabetes checklist**

Answer YES (score 3) if true frequently or most of the time, SOMETIMES (score 2) if true three or more times a month, and SELDOM (score 1) if less than three times a month but more than three times a year. Score 0 if less than that.

Have you noticed any of the following changes in yourself:

1 Do you find yourself excessively thirsty for no obvious reason?
2 Do you pass urine more often but do not have a bladder infection?
3 Has your appetite increased without a change in your activity levels?
4 Have you (in conjunction with any of the above) lost a lot of weight unrelated to a slimming diet?
5 Are you often excessively tired for no apparent reason (late nights etc), and also have any of the above symptoms?

If you answer YES to questions 1 or 2, or to any two of the above, consult the doctor. Meanwhile do NOT go on any diet or do aerobic exercises.

● **Hypoglycaemia checklist**

This is the opposite of diabetes, but often results from similar dietary patterns. Answer and score as for diabetes.

1 Are you very tired first thing in the morning before breakfast?
2 Do you feel edgy, light-headed and shaky when you miss meals or cannot snack and does food ease this?
3 Do you crave sugar-rich foods?
4 Do you depend on stimulants, such as coffee, tea, cola, chocolate, alcohol or cigarettes to give you a "boost" during the day?

If you answered YES to any of these, or SOME-TIMES to more than one, you may be hypogly-caemic. The detox diet and programme will help enormously but eat little and often – up to six times a day. Take six brewer's yeast tablets (a source of chromium which helps sugar metabol-ism) daily with meals (but not if you score high in the Candida questions below). If you answered YES to two or more take professional advice before starting on the detox programme.

● **Candida checklist**

1 Have you taken antibiotics for more than eight weeks or, for shorter periods, four times or more?
2 Have you ever had treatment which involved use of a steroid drug?
3 Have you ever taken "the pill" for a year or more?
4 Have you had more than one preg-nancy, not necessarily to full-term?
5 Have you had vaginal or oral thrush?
6 Have you had endometriosis, persistent or recurrent urethritis, cystitis, vaginitis, or prostatitis?
7 Have you had a fungal skin or nail infec-tion (e.g. athletes foot)?
8 Do you have a variety of allergies or extreme sensitivity to e.g. perfumes, chemicals, tobacco smoke?
9 Do you frequently suffer from long-lasting bowel disorders?
10 Do you crave sweet foods or alcohol, and are your symptoms (e.g. bloating) often worse after eating these?

If you have at least one answer YES in the first four questions, and two or more in the last six, then you probably have an overgrowth of the yeast Candida albicans (see p.38).

Consult a health professional for specific advice on how to control Candida. Follow warn-ings given in the programme about which foods to avoid.

● **Cardiovascular disease**

Anyone over 40 should have a physical checkup before starting the aerobic part of the programme. The following questions should be answered YES (score 3), if the event described occurs once a week or more. Answer SOMETIMES (score 2) if less than weekly but at least three times in the last month and SELDOM (score 1) if less than that but at least six times in the past year.

1 On effort (walking, going upstairs) do you feel either: numb or tingling arm; choking sensation or tightness in neck; pressure sensation in chest or throat; pain in the jaw, throat, neck, shoulder or arm?

2 Do you experience extreme shortness of breath accompanied by feeling faint, weak, and/or exhausted, or have difficulty in breathing when lying down (often associated with swollen ankles or feet)?

3 Do you sometimes experience sudden palpitations, shortness of breath, chest-pain and/or feeling faint, not associated with any effort?

If you answered YES, SOMETIMES or SELDOM to any of these questions you should seek professional advice before starting on the detox programme.

● **Pregnancy**

If you are pregnant, take advice from your health care professional before following the aerobic or dietary aspects of the detox programme.

Allergy and toxicity

These questions will identify people who need to start the detox programme slowly because they are suffering from either an allergy or a reaction to toxic substances. Allergic reactions tend to be intermittent and unpredictable, whereas toxic reactions are either constant or occur at regular intervals. Create three columns: YES-intermittent answers; YES-constant; and NO.

1 Are there dark circles under your eyes?
2 Is your nose stuffed up or runny?
3 Do you have hay fever or asthma?
4 Are your eyes often inflamed or red?
5 Do you have noises in your head?
6 Does your hair come out in clumps?
7 Do you have soaking sweats at night unrelated to hot temperatures?
8 Is your appetite usually poor?
9 Do you get unnatural feelings of sleepiness?
10 Do you pass blood with your stools?
11 Have you liver or gall bladder problems or have you had jaundice?
12 Do you find it difficult to concentrate or think?
13 Are your joints painful, inflamed or swollen?
14 Do you have depression and exhaustion feelings which vanish at weekends and at holiday time?
15 Are you bothered by skin irritation, itching, rashes or hives?
16 Do you get severe headaches for no obvious reason?
17 Are you frequently dizzy or faint?
18 Have you lost interest in sex (unrelated to emotional stress)?
19 Do your eyes often water for no apparent reason?
20 Do you feel tense and jumpy most of the time?

21 Do you have pain or difficulty with uri-
    nating?
22 Are you aware of an itchy sensation in
    your nose and mouth?
23 Do you have periods of unaccountable
    exhaustion, not improved by rest?
24 Are you considered (or do you consider
    yourself) a "sickly" person?
25 Do you have frequent nosebleeds?
26 Are you very underweight?
27 Are you very overweight?
28 Do you have a metallic taste in your
    mouth?
29 Have you ever been treated for cancer?
30 As a child, did you have rheumatic
    fever?
31 Do you suffer from any psychiatric ill-
    ness which is being treated?
32 Are you receiving treatment for any
    chronic illness?
33 Do you feel nausea and often vomit
    after eating?
34 Do you have chronic constipation?
35 Does physical activity of any sort leave
    you totally exhausted?
36 Do you have numb, trembling sensa-
    tions in your hands and feet?
37 Are you considered hyperactive, unable
    to sit still?
38 Do you have muscle spasms and
    cramps and/or muscle tics?
39 Have you lost either your sense of taste
    or of smell?
40 Do you have severe, pus-filled acne?

Score 3 points for every YES. If your overall total
is more than 15, start with the Modified programme, p.86 and then repeat this questionnaire. Do not start the more intensive detox programmes until your score is below 15.

If your anwers suggest you are suffering from
an allergy, get professional advice before you
start a detox programme. If you suspect a toxic
reaction, read the section on the environment
p.113-30. With such symptoms (allergy or toxicity), associated problems, such as fatigue, mental confusion and difficulty in concentrating, fluid
retention, weight fluctuations, muscle and joint
aches and pains, periodic racing pulse, digestive
symptoms, food cravings or skin reactions (urticaria) are common.

If you answered YES to questions 30 or 35 do
not do any aerobic exercises without professional advice, but follow the rest of the programme.

If you answered YES to question 13 avoid
vigorous exercise until you have the advice of a
doctor, osteopath, or chiropractor.

If you answered YES to question 15 take care
with skin brushing not to irritate the skin or any
varicose veins.

If you answered YES to question 10 avoid the
use of enemas and see a doctor.

If you answered YES to question 11 start on
the Modified programme, p.86, as a more intensive detox programme could overload your liver.
See p.182 for coffee enemas and use them
when you feel nauseous.

If you answered YES to questions 21, 29, 31
or 32 do not do any of the dietetic or aerobic
exercise portions of the programmes without
the permission of your doctor. All other aspects
are fine.

PART TWO

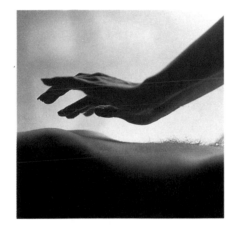

Which programme?

Now that you have worked through the questionnaires –
and answered ALL the questions – you are in a position to
take both a local and a general view of the results:
○ You will have been given local advice where individual
answers required specific remedial action; sometimes you
will also have been given advice if groups of answers led to
intermediate scores (see box on facing page). Never disre-
gard recommendations to seek medical advice or about
which programme to take. Remember you are doing this for
your health.
○ You will now be able to total up a cumulative score
produced by answering all the questionnaires.
     This cumulative score is your key to deciding where to
start detoxifying. At this point you have a preliminary choice
of three dietary detoxification programmes – Ten-day,
Thirty-day, or Modified – and a Basic programme of bodywork techniques. These choices may seem a bit complicated at first, but do not be put off.
     If your cumulative score was above 135, you will first
need to apply the Modified Dietary Detoxification Programme, p.86, for one month and then rework the questionnaires. Only if your score is then below 135 should you
proceed with either the Ten-day or Thirty-day Dietary Detoxification Programmes. This cautiousness is necessary
because such a level of toxicity in your life is sufficiently high
to warrant extra care in detoxification, and taking the process in two stages. When your total score is under 135, you
may safely proceed to choosing between Ten-day or Thirty-
day Detox programmes. The intensive Ten-day Dietary
Detoxification Programme, p.74, demands that you stop
work, be able to rest and not drive during the whole period.
If this is not possible, or if you in any case prefer to, choose
the more leisurely Thirty-day Dietary Detoxification Programme, p.80.
     Whichever dietary detox programme you embark on, you
will need to combine it with the Basic programme of
bodywork techniques, p.62. This introduces you to the first
steps in breathing and relaxation techniques, a start in the
use of hydrotherapy methods, introductory stretching exercises and an explanation of what is involved in aerobic
exercise. You also begin to use massage methods which
encourage circulatory and lymphatic function. The Basic
programme prepares your body for the more advanced
methods of Maintenance (Part 3).
     The Maintenance programme describes normal daily liv-

ing – a life plan in which diet, patterns of exercise, rest and mental hygiene are arranged on a sustainable basis to govern a future of high-level health and vitality. It builds on the work done in the Ten-day or Thirty-day Dietary Detox programmes, and on the Basic programme.

Follow Basic for the first ten days of detoxification, then introduce techniques from Maintenance, though leaving its advanced meditation, visualization and autogenic-training methods for a further ten days until you have learned to relax enough to do them. Practise instead the Basic relaxation methods. After Day 20, all complementary bodywork techniques will be from the Maintenance programme. The flowcharts on pp.74-5 and 80-1 will help you to deal with all this detail.

If you started with Modified Dietary Detox to begin with, you will be using all the exercise techniques from Maintenance by the time you finish. When you move to the more intensive dietary programmes, continue with them and do NOT go back to Basic methods.

It is recommended that once or twice a year, you rework the questionnaires, re-evaluate your score and, if necessary, go through one of the dietary detox programmes again. Again, do not return to Basic, but continue with the bodywork technique levels reached in Maintenance.

Drugs p.48
If the total score of the four sections (alcohol, smoking, caffeine and medicinal drugs) is above 20, do not start either Ten- or Thirty-day Dietary Detoxification Programmes. Go to Modified, p.86, for at least six weeks; rework the questionnaire and rescore.

Diet, p.50-1
Individual deficiencies which might be associated with symptoms described are indicated in the text. Reassess these after detoxification and see which have improved. Those which have not will need specific supplementation.

If the total score in this section is above 50, you need to pay extra special attention to your diet. The programmes themselves will help with this, of course, and the questions in each of these sections will guide you towards corrective action for particular aspects of your toxicity.

Ailments, p.52-3
If your score is above 15, start with the Modified programme, p.86. Only go to the other detox programmes when your score is below 15.

Overall score
If your overall score (including totals for Ailments and Dietary factors and Drugs) is above 135, start with the Modified programme, p.86. Rescore to assess whether you have come below 135 and are therefore ready for the basic dietary detox programmes.

Preparing to detox

The fact that you are reading this book probably means that you are dissatisfied with your present condition; that you want a higher level of health which allows you to realize your full potential and gives you a better quality of life. Even so, you may feel strongly tempted to quit after a few days on the detox programme. As your body attempts to clear substances that have lain hidden for years, you may experience signs of toxic overload, such as nausea, lethargy, or flu-like symptoms. You will need to be strong in your motivation, determined in your desire for better health and assertive in your attitude, so that you recognize these changes for what they are: positive steps towards your goal. Ask yourself:

* Do you know why you are doing this?
* Do you want to be as healthy as you are able to be?
* Do you want to clear your system of the toxic wastes that have sapped your energy and vitality for so long?
* Are you tired of being tired, sick of being sick?
* And, most importantly, do you understand what is being asked of you – what detoxification entails?

If so, read on as you push on into the programmes themselves. Get ready for action.

Make sure that the environment in which you will spend your time on the detox programmes is wholesome, pleasant and free of toxins.

1 Stock up on all the ingredients beforehand. Read the dietary instructions carefully, before you begin, and go shopping for what you will need.
2 Make a wall chart of the instructions with times and details of all the interacting factors. Include aspects of the Basic programme and the taking of supplements.
3 Have good reading material to hand, music to listen to, and materials for any hobbies you enjoy.
4 Ask friends not to phone, or else disconnect the phone altogether.
5 Sleep as much as your body wants to; it may be a surprising amount.
6 Listen to the radio, and be selective about what you watch on TV, since negative images can upset you.
7 Place an ionizer where you will spend most time (see p.114); get a natural-fibre mat or futon for exercising on.
8 Avoid taking proprietary medication during this period, unless absolutely essential (see p. 60–1).
9 Keep a diary of your dreams. Later they may begin to make sense to you.
10 Remember that you are doing something of great value for your body; that you are creating an oasis of cleansing and calm within which it can regenerate. Know you are in control and have chosen a path that leads to improved health.

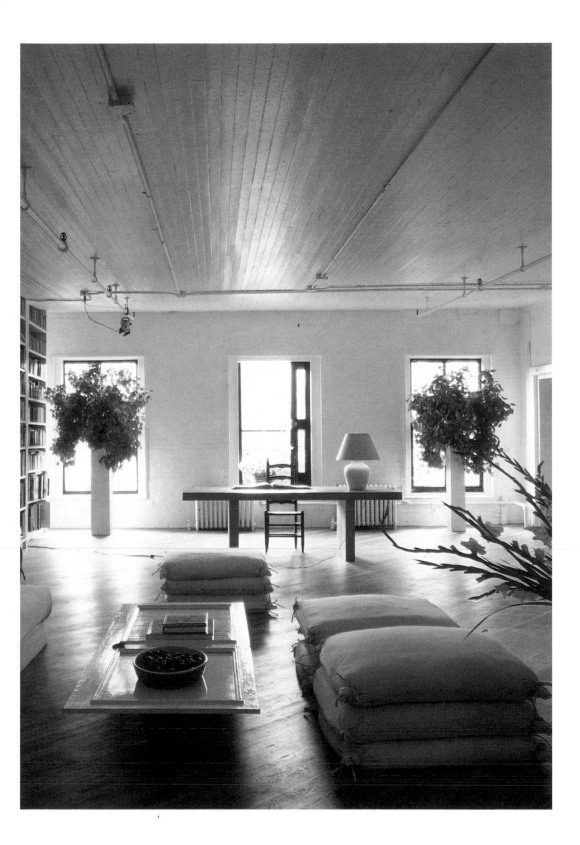

Side effects

As you detoxify, the main organs involved have to cope with rather more than their regular daily tasks and this can produce a variety of harmless, if somewhat annoying, symptoms. Many of these symptoms are nothing more than evidence of detoxification in action. There is, however, a great deal you can do to reduce most such symptoms without suppressing the detoxification process itself. The severity and number of symptoms is related to how many toxins are released into your system as detoxification starts. If your initial level of toxicity is high, or if you choose a rapid detoxification technique such as fasting, more of these toxic wastes are released and therefore the greater the number and severity of the symptoms. As you become less toxic you will have fewer symptoms during intensive detoxification and eventually they will stop altogether.

Use the safe symptom treatments described on this page and elsewhere, but do not use drugs, even aspirin, without expert guidance; the body reacts more violently to drugs during detoxification.

Cold
Because you will be eating less, and most of your available energy will be diverted to the detoxification process, you may feel colder than usual. Deal with this simply by wearing more clothes or turning up the heating in your home. Take extra care after exercising, hydrotherapy, or baths and showers, not to get chilled.

Headache
One of the most common side-effects of detoxification and fasting is a headache. These usually appear during the first 48 hours of detoxification. To alleviate a detox headache use the acupressure points de-scribed on p.73 and/or trigger point methods (p.181) and/or a cold compress and/or a coffee enema (p.182). The coffee enema can usually clear a "sick" headache or migraine too.

Nausea
You may feel nauseous in the early stages of detoxification, especially while fasting. A hos-pital-based study in Belfast has shown how this unpleasant sensation can be relieved by applying pressure to a point above the wrist (p.73) for one minute as often as necessary.

A method that deals with the toxic build-up which causes nausea, is the coffee enema (p.182). Coffee taken this way goes directly to the liver and stimulates that organ to rapidly excrete copious amounts of tox-in-containing bile. This re-lieves the liver considerably and eases symptoms. You can use it many times a day, until the toxic reaction fades.

Concentration
In the early stages of detoxifica-tion, or while fasting, you may find it difficult to focus your attention for any length of time. Make sure you get plenty of rest, listen to music or the radio and spend only short periods trying to cope with any-thing that demands concentra-tion. Above all DO NOT drive or use dangerous machinery or equipment.

● **Bowel health**

During the early stages of the detox programme, bowel health and function may, in a very few individuals, be affected. Do not, therefore, become too concerned if either diarrhoea or constipation develop. Only if these become severely uncomfortable should you consider doing or taking anything to "force" the body to alter its process of adaptation. Your homoeostatic, self- regulating machinery will usually normalize such problems without help.

The regular supplementation of friendly bacteria such as Lactobacillus acidophilus or bifidobacteria for some weeks before starting a detoxification programme make such reactions as diarrhoea or constipation far less likely.

● **Constipation**

This may occur because of a rapid increase in fluid loss (such as urination or sweating) and inadequate fluid intake as you begin to make desirable changes in your diet and exercise pattern. It may also just be the result of your bowels getting used to these new foods.

Follow the guidelines given (p.133) for fluid intake, and eat slowly and chew thoroughly. Your reformed dietary pattern will ultimately ensure that adequate fibre is taken in and the problem will disappear within a few days. Use enemas as directed during fasting (see p.182).

● **Diarrhoea**

It is not unusual after a few days of detoxification for the bowels to become very loose and watery. This should cause no concern as it is usually evidence of the rapid elimination of undesirable substances. Make sure that you take additional liquid in the form of spring water or potassium broth (p.76). If diarrhoea persists for more than three days take professional advice.

Weight loss
Not surprisingly, when you reduce your food intake, weight loss is likely. In the early stages surplus liquid is shed, often leading to a drop of several pounds in the first day or so. After the first few days, however, weight loss tends to slow down and becomes more gradual. As you become detoxified and healthy, your weight will tend to adjust to what is correct for your body type, taking into account energy output and age.

Rashes
During detoxification the skin has to cope with large quantities of wastes coming through it. This can result in rashes and blemishes at first. Cope with this by stringent hygienic care: bathe frequently and change underwear often. Use skin friction (p.66), salt glow (p.161), oatmeal and essential oil baths (p.162), peat baths (p.163), a face sauna or green clay applications (p.165) to keep the skin soothed and pores open.

Amino acids for vegetarians

Vegetarians have better health, on the whole, than people who eat meat. However, they only achieve this benefit if they pay scrupulous attention to getting enough of the basic elements of protein, (called amino acids) from vegetables or dairy products (see p.85). Vegetarians tend to have smaller reserves of fat and "spare" protein than meat eaters; they probably also have a lesser degree of dietary toxicity. During periods of strict detoxification, therefore, if you are vegetarian, and average or slightly underweight for your height, take between 10 and 15 grams of a balanced formulation of the full spectrum of free form amino acids daily. These supplements should contain at least the eight essential amino acids and ideally all twenty amino acids that the body uses to make protein. Take them between meals with water.

Basic programme

Whichever dietary detoxification programme is indicated for you, (based on your current level of toxicity and wellbeing, as assessed in the questionnaires on p.44–54), it needs to be complemented by a start on basic introductory techniques involving breathing (p.63), relaxation (p.64), hydrotherapy (p.66), stretching (p.68), aerobic exercise (p.70) and massage (p.71).

Detailed explanations of these methods are given on the following pages, and it is most important that you carefully apply all of them, in each case following the guidelines before eventually moving on to the more advanced approaches in the Maintenance section (Part 3). The importance of those associated methods and modalities will become clearer as you progress towards the full detoxification programme.

In each case the physical detoxification method, e.g. hydrotherapy or massage, is valuable in itself or as an aid to reducing the mental and physical tensions which slow down detoxification.

A graduated progression is needed in most instances so as to avoid undue physical stress. As an example: you will find that in order to achieve deep relaxation, itself an essential precursor to meditation, you must first learn to breathe freely and deeply. Similarly, if you are going to achieve both the physical and mental detox benefits of aerobic exercise, it is vital that you not only follow the aerobics explanation, but also perform the regular stretching exercises outlined.

The objective of detoxification is vital health and wellbeing. As you embark on this journey, have these goals firmly in mind, for there are very few shortcuts and the methods and exercises in the Basic programme are your necessary first steps. The route is well signposted and the map is in your hands.

Breathing

Learning to breathe with attention can bring a wide variety of benefits. Breathing both oxygenates the blood and acts to eliminate unwanted wastes from the body. It therefore plays an important part in chemical detoxification, but, in addition to this, it also helps you to release emotional and stress-induced tensions.

Unless breathing is rhythmic and slow it is impossible to relax, either physically or mentally. Most people use only part of their breathing capacity, and many breathe extremely badly, causing quite serious health problems. These exercises (and the stretching and aerobic exercises on p.68-70) encourage normal breathing function. Do not dismiss them as unimportant; though simple they will prepare you for the more advanced versions in Maintenance, p.149 and also produce a sense of relaxation.

Aim to get into a pattern of doing the breathing exercises regularly, ideally twice a day, perhaps before two of your meals. This will fix a time for them in the day so that they become part of your life routine. If at all possible do the exercises in fresh air; when indoors try to have windows open. Make sure your clothing is not restrictive, preventing the free movement of the ribs and chest muscles.

Breathing exercises
Practise your breathing exercises at least once, and ideally twice, a day for at least five minutes each time. Do them in a calm, unhurried atmosphere, so the obvious mechanical advantage of deep breathing is also accompanied by a chance for relaxation. Always breathe in through your nose and exhale through your mouth. Repeat each exercise 15 times. When you have finished, make sure that you take a few minutes rest or you may feel slightly dizzy.

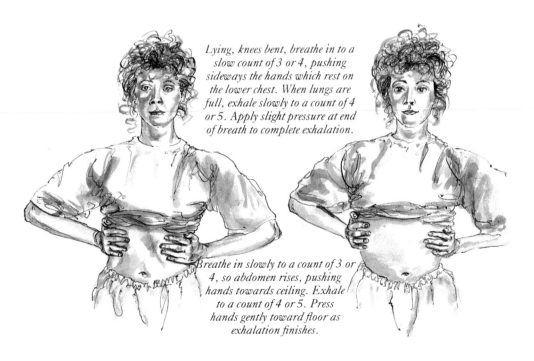

Lying, knees bent, breathe in to a slow count of 3 or 4, pushing sideways the hands which rest on the lower chest. When lungs are full, exhale slowly to a count of 4 or 5. Apply slight pressure at end of breath to complete exhalation.

Breathe in slowly to a count of 3 or 4, so abdomen rises, pushing hands towards ceiling. Exhale to a count of 4 or 5. Press hands gently toward floor as exhalation finishes.

Relaxation

We now know that the mind is in complete control of the immune system, the body's defence mechanisms. In order to achieve physical detoxification it is also necessary for your mind to become calm, and the first step toward this is to relax the muscles of the body. Most of us, to a greater or lesser extent, unconsciously hold our muscles in a state of unnecessary tension. This tension prevents the mind from becoming truly still and, because the muscles use more energy than any other body system, it leads to an enormous waste of energy, and symptoms such as fatigue, stiffness, aches, and pains.

In these exercises you will first be asked to contract strongly and then relax all areas of your body in sequence, sensing the difference between the states of tension and relaxation. When a muscle is strongly contracted a strange, but perfectly normal, reaction occurs: it is obliged, through nervous-system activity, to become more relaxed than it was before the contraction. The purpose of the exercise is to make you familiar with the sensation of deep relaxation, thus teaching you to relax to an ever greater extent. This prepares you for more advanced relaxation techniques in the Maintenance programme (p.102).

Progressive relaxation
Do these exercises at the same time every day, in a warm room with a calm, unhurried atmosphere. Wear loose clothing.

The captions describe the sequence and explain how to tense each area but do not repeat the tensing/relaxing technique each time.

This technique involves first tensing the area described strongly for five seconds, then tensing even harder for a few seconds more, before releasing totally. Then spend five seconds savouring the sense of relaxation thus produced. This technique must be used for every part of the sequence, every time you are told to work on a particular area.

Lie comfortably, without stiffness, legs outstretched, arms by your side. Focus on your right foot and lower leg. Tense these by bringing your toes toward your face. Follow the sequence described above; then repeat with your left leg. Then tense each leg the other way, curling the toes under and tightening the muscles at the back of the leg.

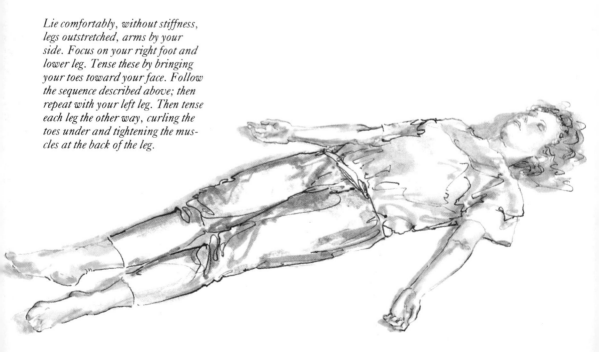

BEWARE: if you wear contact
lenses DO NOT do any exercises which screw up the eyes.

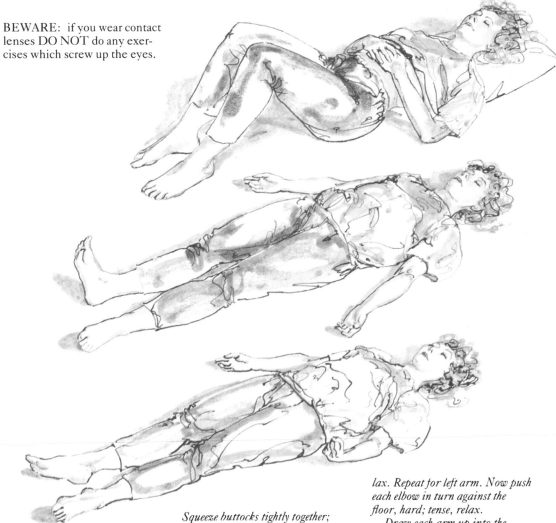

Tense the muscles round the
kneecap strongly as though pulling
the kneecap toward the hip. Next
tense the muscles behind the knee by
pushing it down against the floor.
Do each leg in turn.

Strongly contract the buttock
and thigh muscles that draw your
leg toward your hip. Do both sides.
right and left. Complete by pushing
each leg strongly away from you.

Squeeze buttocks tightly together;
tense, relax. Draw lower abdomen
in tightly, tense, relax; push it up
toward the ceiling. Push lower
back hard against the floor, then
arch it up toward the ceiling. Always follow sequence on p.64.
Work on upper torso the same way.

Clench each hand in turn into a
fist; tense, relax. Now stretch each
hand, holding fingers as far out as
possible.

Now hold your right elbow up,
tense arm rigidly, release and re-

lax. Repeat for left arm. Now push
each elbow in turn against the
floor, hard; tense, relax.

Draw each arm up into the
shoulder, holding it stiff, increase
tension, release and relax. Now
stretch each arm in turn with equal
force. Increase tension, release,
relax.

To relax the neck, tighten the
muscles as much as you can. Tense
more, release, relax. To finish,
relax the all-important facial muscles. Purse your lips tightly, or
open your mouth as wide as you
can, using the tensing/relaxing
technique.

Hydrotherapy

The skin is one of the main routes used by your body to eliminate toxic wastes. The blood system transports wastes via small capillaries to its surface, where they are eliminated through the skin pores. The outer surface, however, is made up of "dead" cells, which along with any accumulated oils and microscopic dirt particles can seriously reduce the efficiency of this major cleansing organ. Hydrotherapy (or water-treatment) methods increase the local circulation of blood to the skin, and also clear away surface debris. In this way they improve elimination by speeding up delivery of wastes and unblocking the pores. In addition, they markedly improve overall skin tone and quality, and also help to mobilize unsightly deposits of fat and waste material (cellulite) lying underneath the skin.

To have any real impact on what may be a long-standing problem of sluggish circulation and elimination, this work must be done regularly. Establish a pattern of a good skin-brushing at least every other day, with either an Epsom salt bath or trunk pack on intervening days. Aim to have at least one Epsom salt bath and one trunk pack a week, and ideally two, but never have more than two Epsom salt baths in any one week.

Skin brushing
Do this before washing while your skin is still dry. It takes a few minutes to brush – rub the main areas of the body carefully – firmly, but not enough to irritate the skin. Anticipate a good "red" reaction, indicating circulatory response, along with a fantastic glow. If using a loofah, bath-mit, or brush, rub with a circular "creeping" motion to avoid rubbing in one place too much. Using a towel has a weaker "red" effect but will not irritate sensitive areas as much. Give most attention to the back, the legs and arms. After a week the skin will be less sensitive and more pressure can be used; but start gently for best results.

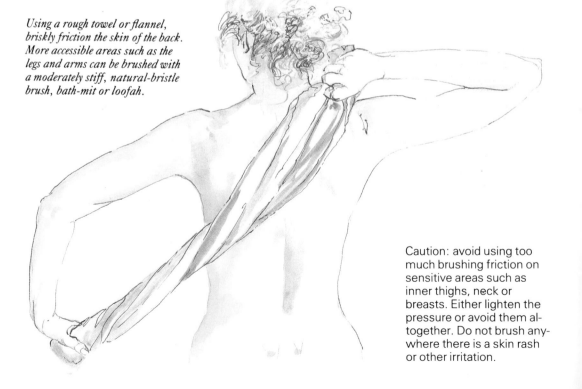

Using a rough towel or flannel, briskly friction the skin of the back. More accessible areas such as the legs and arms can be brushed with a moderately stiff, natural-bristle brush, bath-mit or loofah.

Caution: avoid using too much brushing friction on sensitive areas such as inner thighs, neck or breasts. Either lighten the pressure or avoid them altogether. Do not brush anywhere there is a skin rash or other irritation.

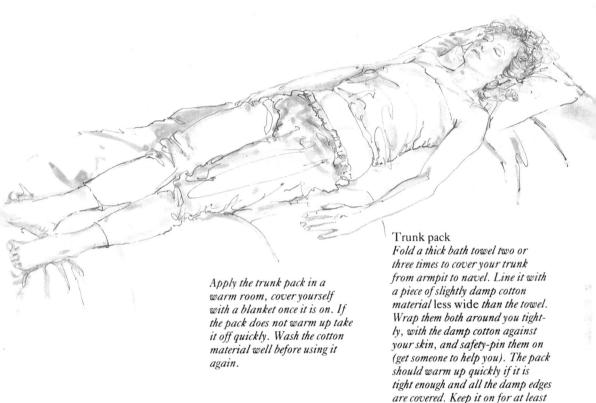

Apply the trunk pack in a warm room, cover yourself with a blanket once it is on. If the pack does not warm up take it off quickly. Wash the cotton material well before using it again.

Trunk pack
Fold a thick bath towel two or three times to cover your trunk from armpit to navel. Line it with a piece of slightly damp cotton material less wide than the towel. Wrap them both around you tightly, with the damp cotton against your skin, and safety-pin them on (get someone to help you). The pack should warm up quickly if it is tight enough and all the damp edges are covered. Keep it on for at least half an hour.

Epsom salt bath
This increases elimination through the skin dramatically, but you certainly cannot wash in it. Place between half a pound and a pound of commercial Epsom salt and quarter pound of sea salt in a hot bath. Stay in this for not less than ten and not more than twenty minutes, topping up the hot water throughout. Get out and dry yourself quickly before getting into a preheated bed. You will probably sweat profusely and sleep deeply. Have some drinking water by the bed to make up for lost liquid, and apply a natural moisturizer to your skin the next morning.

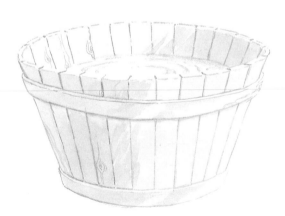

CAUTION: Epsom salt baths are not recommended for anyone with eczema or high blood pressure.

Stretching

Your daily activities at work, in sport, and hobbies, your postural habits, and the tensions that build up through emotional reactions, can all act to increase the stiffness (or tone) of your muscles. High muscle tone can be an advantage when accompanied by flexibility, but in many adults it may be unnecessarily high, leading to chronic shortening of the muscles and problems such as slowing down the flow of lymph.

Lymph is a general waste-disposal medium that carries cellular debris for reprocessing and elimination. The flow of lymph depends on the action of several "body pumps" such as the alternating pressures caused by breathing, and the contraction and relaxation of muscles as they work. This action is diminished if muscle tone is permanently high. Also, the muscles are major users of energy, and excess tone is wasteful of this commodity. Regular stretching works on both these problems, thus helping detoxification. Increased flexibility also makes you less liable to strains and sprains when you start more active exercise. Try to do these exercises daily and never less than every other day. Always do them before aerobic exercises. Don't do them too soon after a meal.

CAUTION: if you have a back problem or arthritis, check with your medical adviser before doing these exercises.
 Never do them to the point of pain.
 They are not contraindicated if you are pregnant.

Back stretch
This exercise stretches most of the muscles on the back of the body from the neck to the lower leg. If you find it difficult to do it as illustrated, sit on your heels, knees bent, and stretch forward from there, forehead to floor, arms outstretched). The method shown below, however, is much more effective.

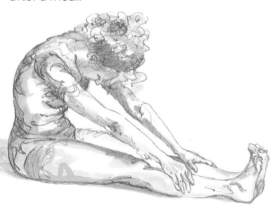

Sit with both legs straight, toes up, and bend forward. Grasp one leg with each hand, forehead toward knees. Hold this for half a minute. Exhaling, try to stretch forward another inch. Hold for a few seconds.

Sit with one leg straight, the other bent, as shown in the illustration. Exhaling, bend forward and grasp straight leg with both hands, inclining forehead toward your knee. Hold for 30 seconds, breathing deeply and slowly, and then stretch a bit more as you exhale. Hold a few seconds. Switch legs; repeat.

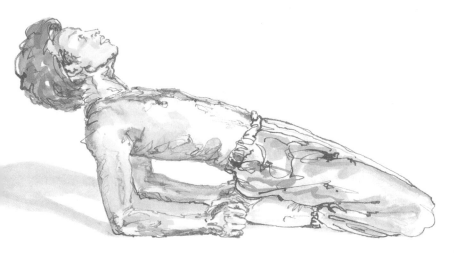

Front stretch and back-arch
These exercises stretch the front of the thighs and the trunk, as well as loosening different parts of the rib cage. This helps encourage normal breathing. As with all stretching exercises, make sure that, as you release your breath, you relax slightly further into the stretch. In the Maintenance section (p.154) other exercises will be added to these basic stretching movements.

Sit on your heels, your hands on the floor behind you. Exhaling, arch your back so your lower abdomen and pelvis are pushed forward, head backward. Hold this for 30 seconds, breathing deeply.

Now bend your elbows and lie back, resting your weight on your forearms. In this position arch your back and pelvis upward taking your head backward and hold for three breathing cycles (half a minute).

Crouch on your hands and knees, with your thighs at right angles to the floor. Your hands should be flat and pointing forward, and your head hanging down. Exhaling, arch your back upward, pulling in the abdomen. Hold for at least five deep breathing cycles trying to breathe into your arched back. You should feel a pull on your neck, upper arms and rounded back.

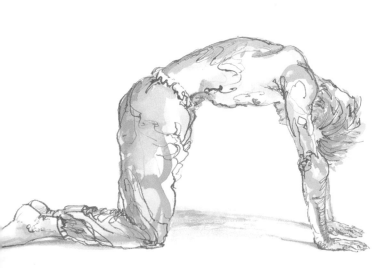

CAUTION: you may feel a bit giddy after the deep breathing which these exercises call for. To avoid this, sit quietly for a minute or so, breathing normally, when you have finished before standing up again.

Aerobic exercise

Aerobic exercise is any physical activity that increases your heart rate above the level at which it easily copes, and keeps it there for at least twenty minutes. As and when you repeatedly reach this training level, your cardiovascular function improves, so you need to make more effort (train harder or for longer) to get the heart (pulse) rate up to the required level. With this improvement in circulation and oxygenation, your ability to detoxify increases.

The amount and intensity of exercise needed for an aerobic effect differs from person to person and changes as you get fitter. So it is necessary first to establish your individual pulse indicators and, second, periodically to re-assess these figures.

The form of exercise you choose is limited only by the requirement that it raise your pulse to the right level for long enough. Brisk walking is as good as any and far safer than jogging, which can jar weight-bearing joints if you are not already fit. Make sure you have good supporting training shoes and wear an appropriate tracksuit or sweatshirt. Aerobic exercise should be done three times a week to achieve a training effect. (See also p.150 and p.156.)

Exercise variations
Use any form of exercise that takes your pulse rate above your base pulse level (see below). This can be cycling, swimming (though it is very hard to get aerobic effect without heroic effort), jogging (be careful of your knees and ankles), trampoline, skipping, dancing, or, of course, aerobic classes. The safest is walking.

Wrist: look for your pulse about an inch above the wrist crease on the thumb side of either forearm. Arterial pulse: feel lightly, just in front of the muscle which runs down from behind your ear to your collar bone, about an inch and a half below your jaw-line.

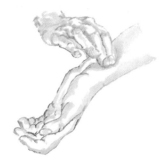
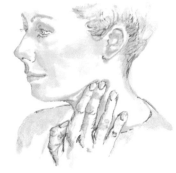

Using one or two fingers count your pulse either at the wrist or neck. Count for 30 seconds and multiply by two for your pulse rate.

Pulse assessment
For three days on waking, record your pulse for one minute and calculate your average morning pulse rate (e.g. 72 + 68 + 70 = 210 ÷ 3 = 70). Add this number to your age and subtract the total from 220 (220 − (70 + e.g.40) = 110). Find 60% and 80% of this result (= 66 and 88). Now add back your morning average: 66 + 70 = 136, and 88 + 70 = 158. This gives you two very important numbers. Remember your own numbers are unique and variable according to your age and pulse rate.

To have any aerobic effect you have to increase your pulse rate above the smaller number (136 in our example) for at least 20 minutes, three times a week, while keeping it below the higher number (158) to avoid straining your heart. Check your pulse rate regularly while exercising to keep it within range. As you get fitter, and as you get older, your morning pulse rate will drop so you will have to recalculate these numbers from time to time and work to the new values.

Massage

Massage can be both relaxing and extremely helpful to detoxification. The mechanical movement of lymph and blood through the muscles which good massage achieves, enhances the efficiency of all the other things that you will be doing to improve these functions, such as stretching exercises, hydrotherapy and aerobics. Nothing can take the place of a professional massage, but the basic strokes described here and on p.171, are quite easy to learn. Once you have done so, you can exchange massages with your partner. This is particularly desirable during the detoxification process and at times of stress.

The requirements are few: a warm comfortable room and a surface on which to work, such as a futon or mattress; time to give or receive the massage without hurry (not less than half an hour and ideally nearer an hour), and an intent made up of a combination of caring, affection, and nurturing which is possibly even more important than the techniques themselves. Get a lotion, oil or cream suitable for massage from herbal suppliers, health store, body shop or pharmacy. Choose one with only natural ingredients. Choice of oil or lotion is a personal matter (lotion, being less slippery, allows more control) and does alter the effectiveness of the massage. Some massage oils now have essential oils added to them, which are both aromatically pleasant and can encourage circulatory or skin function. Try to have a massage at least once, and ideally two or three times, a week.

How to massage
Your hands need to be relaxed, warm, and firm. Avoid hurried, aimless contacts. "Mould" your hands to the area you touch and hold in your mind the intention to help, to relax, and to nurture. Vary the pressure depending on the receiver's sensitivity (no pain should be felt) and what you want to achieve. Use enough lotion or oil so the hands glide on the skin without dragging, but not so much that you lose control over the strokes.

The tissues between the neck and shoulders, the buttocks, low back, calf, or arm muscles, can be relaxed and stretched by a series of wringing actions. One hand gently grasps a handful of muscle, lifting and pulling it toward you as the other pulls it away from you.

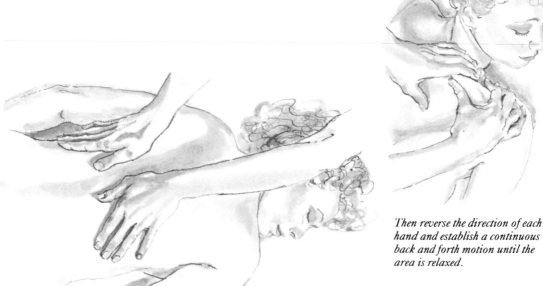

Then reverse the direction of each hand and establish a continuous back and forth motion until the area is relaxed.

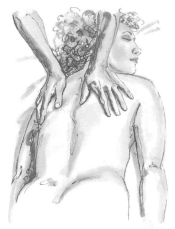

Start at the base of the neck, with the heels of your hands alongside the spine, fingers pointing down and slightly outward. Use the stroking technique. Then move your hands slightly outward, away from the spine and repeat the stroke, until the upper back feels relaxed and warm.

Stroking technique
Mould your hands to the tissue and stroke symmetrically away from yourself. After 12 inches, fan out and circle back to the starting position. Repeat. The main contact is with the heel and palm of the hand.

Next apply the stroking technique from the level where the previous strokes ended and circle outward at waist level. Cover all the muscles at the side of the spine in this way.

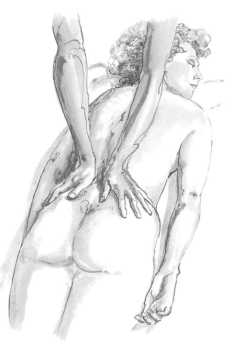

Now apply the same stroke to the area from the waist down to the buttocks. Fan out at that level to stroke across and down, toward the hips.

*   When the lower back feels warm, treat the buttock and shoulder areas to a series of gentle wringing strokes. Finish with some light caressing moves to relax everything that has been worked on.*

Acupressure
Pressure on reflex areas on the
body surface can safely be used
to achieve some remarkable
effects. The points illustrated
are useful during detoxification
and specifically to reduce feelings of nausea, including both
morning and sea-sickness. Self-
applied thumb pressure should
never cause pain when these
points are firmly pressed for 30
to 60 seconds. If necessary, as
in the nausea point, they can
be treated many times each day
without harm.

*The point Pericardium 6 is found
on the palmer surface of the forearm, two widths of your thumb
towards the elbow from the wrist
crease, between the tendons. Press
this for up to a minute at a time
whenever you feel a sense of
nausea, a common symptom in the
early stages of detoxification. This
point is now used in major hospitals in the UK for self-treatment of
morning sickness.*

*The point Stomach 36 is used to
balance digestive and eliminative
functions and to enhance energy. It
is found the width of your three
middle fingers below the lower level
of the knee cap, in a hollow just in
front of the upper aspect of the
fibula (the small bone on the outside of the lower leg). Press this on
either leg for up to a minute some
time before your main meals.*

*Large intestine point 4 is in the
fleshy region between your thumb
and index finger. Careful probing
with your other thumb will locate it
as a sensitive area. Press this gently for up to a minute shortly before
your main meals. This also helps
to relieve headaches.*

Ten-day dietary detoxification programme

If you have decided to detoxify rapidly, check that your score in the questionnaires confirms this is a suitable choice (refer back to p.56-7 for general guidance).

The Ten-day programme is distinguished almost entirely by a stricter diet than the Thirty-day or Modified programmes. All other elements, such as relaxation methods, massage, hydrotherapy, and exercise, require the Basic programme (p.62-73) of introduction, whatever dietary programme is indicated or chosen. After the Ten-day detox programme you should, therefore, continue using the body-work methods in the Basic programme until you have progressed enough at this level to move on to the more advanced Maintenance programme (Part 3).

Before you start
Read the guidelines on p.58 for preparing for a detox programme. Also prepare a space for doing relaxation and massage. Eat only a light salad or soup on the evening before you start.

Reassess
Periodically repeat the questionnaires to see how much you are improving or if you need to detoxify again. If you do, you could try either of the two dietary detox programmes, Ten-day or Thirty-day.

Day Twenty onwards
If you have practised your relaxation exercises regularly, you should now be ready to move onto the autogenic-training, meditation, and visualization methods described on pp.102-3 and 107-10. All other elements of the Maintenance programme should now be in place. Your level of energy and wellbeing should be considerably enhanced after this initial effort at detoxification.

Days Eleven to Twenty
You should now follow the diet in the Maintenance section on p.131-9, and start using some of its bodywork techniques. But do not modify your relaxation programme for at least another ten days. You may not yet be able to relax sufficiently to use the more advanced methods.

Amino acids

If you are vegetarian, refer to the note on p.61 about amino acid supplements. Take these throughout the Ten-day programme. Also take them if you do not eat dairy produce or cannot ensure the right food combinations (see p.85).

Days One to Two
Start this detox programme with one of the three fasts outlined on p.76. Also begin using the methods in the Basic programme, but avoid doing anything too strenuous. Pay particular attention to hydrother-apy. Rest as much as you can. Read p.60-1 to find out about detox side-effects.

Days Three to Eight
During this time your diet should be mainly raw food (p.77). Prac-tise all the methods in the Basic programme faithfully but do not over-exert yourself. Take any sup-plements recommended on p.76. If you are vegetarian take additional amino acids (see note on this page and on p.61). Conserve your energy, do not become too active.

Day Nine
Eat more complex meals on Day Nine, with more protein at main meals (see p.78-9). Remember to chew thoroughly. If you have a sensitive digestion read about food combining on p.132 and use this to guide your future selections. Con-tinue the Basic bodywork methods.

Day Ten
Increase the amount of protein with your main meals and have the same breakfast as on Day Nine (see p.78-9). You will soon move on to the diet in Maintenance (p.131-9). Continue with all elements of the Basic programme.

Pregnancy caution
Many pregnant women have benefited from the detoxification methods described. However, this sort of programme should never be considered un-less medical clearance is given and adequate super-vision is available.

Diet: Days One and Two

● Menu

For the first two days choose from:

* A water-only fast — undoubtedly the most effective but also the most likely to produce transient unpleasant side-effects (see note below). Use either bottled water or well-filtered tap water since they do not contain impurities.
* A modified fast on fruit, which is detoxifying but not as effective as a water-only fast.
* A "potassium-broth" fast (see recipe below), which uses mineral-rich water. This is an efficient detoxifying method and is also somewhat tastier than water.

Whatever form of fasting you choose, have only a light meal the night before, perhaps a salad, some live yoghurt, a bowl of vegetable soup, or an all-fruit meal.

If you choose the water or broth fast, make sure you do not drink either less than four pints or more than eight pints daily. Drink some liquid every two hours or whenever you feel thirsty. Try to "chew" the liquid, by keeping it in your mouth for some seconds, rather than drinking hastily. If you choose the fruit-fast option, select fruits such as apples, pears, grapes, peaches or papaya. If you wish to juice these, dilute them 50:50 with pure (not tap) water, and sip slowly. Avoid the more allergenic citrus fruits during fasting.

NOTE: To either the water or fruit juice add a quarter teaspoonful of vitamin C (ascorbic acid) powder to each pint of liquid (use calcium or sodium ascorbate obtainable from health stores and pharmacies).

If you are eating the fruit have a little whenever hungry but not more than three pounds per day. Chew well and slowly and also drink at least two pints of water or broth daily.

To ensure that your bowels are cleared while fasting, apply one of the methods below, whether you have had a normal bowel movement that day or not.

* A warm-water enema (see p.182)
* A dose of powdered (not husks of) psyllium seeds (obtainable from health stores). Mix a tablespoon of powder with half a pint of water in a blender and drink it. This bulk is not absorbed, but ensures a clearance of the bowel that attracts toxic wastes during the fast.

NOTE: While on the Ten-day programme take these supplements daily: one high-potency multimineral capsule; one high-potency multivitamin capsule or tablet.

Potassium broth
Place five pints of water in a stainless-steel or pyrex pan. Add four cups of chopped mixed vegetables. Cook on a low heat for half an hour; use no seasoning. Strain the liquid and discard the vegetables. Refrigerate until use.

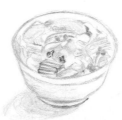

NOTE: See p.60 for an explanation of why symptoms are not always undesirable. Then read p.141 for an explanation of the special symptoms which often accompany fasting/detoxification. See p.73 for acupressure methods of symptom relief.

Days Three to Eight

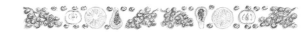

● **Preparing food**

During these intensive detox days avoid spending too much time in the kitchen by preparing the fruit and salads you will eat beforehand. Get them washed, drained, and wrapped in the refrigerator, ready to eat whenever you want (except for the dressing, if required). To steam, suspend the vegetables above boiling water until just tender (three to four minutes). To stir-fry, wipe the pan with oil and stir the vegetables constantly with a wooden spoon for a few minutes, to tenderize but not overcook them (see p.134).

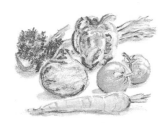

● **Menu**

For breakfast choose:

* Two or three items of: apples, pears, grapes, peaches, papaya, mango, melon, Kiwi fruit, strawberries, blueberries, raspberries, or other berries, orange, grapefruit, or other citrus fruits. Avoid banana or avocado at this meal; and

* *Either* one or two ounces of sunflower or pumpkin seeds, *or* one or two ounces of freshly-shelled walnuts, pecan, hazelnuts, or almonds; and

* Drink *either* a cup of unsweetened herbal tea (see p.138 for a list of safe ones) *or* some lemon juice and hot water with up to half a teaspoon of honey.

For lunch and evening meal choose *either*

* A mixed raw salad of not less than four varieties of salad vegetable with at least one orange/red component (beet, carrot, tomato, red pepper) as well as shredded green ingredients. Try to include items such as parsley, celery, and cress for mineral content. *Or*

* Mixed stir-fried or steamed vegetables (if digestion cannot take raw salads and as an evening meal on alternate days, in rotation with salad).

Combine these with the items below.

At one of the main meals, choose from:

* A baked jacket potato (dressed with olive oil)

* A cupful of boiled, unpolished rice or millet (cooked with onion for flavour)

* One or two bananas

And at the other main meal, choose from:

* An avocado

* Two ounces of cottage cheese

* A poached or boiled egg

* Stir-fried or plain tofu (bean curd from oriental and health stores)

NOTE: Avoid mixtures of concentrated carbohydrates and proteins: do not *at the same meal* eat the carbohydrates in the first block together with the proteins in the second block (Eg, avoid potato plus cheese, or banana plus egg.)

For dessert: a few ounces of live, unsweetened yoghurt, or an apple or pear.

Healthy salad dressing

Avoid vinegar and brand-name dressings. Use pure olive oil and lemon juice (delicious too on lightly cooked or raw vegetables); or add live yoghurt (with a little crushed garlic, if desired) instead. For a subtle flavour, rub a salad bowl with sliced garlic. Try adding mint leaves to salads for additional aroma and taste.

Liquids

Drink at least two pints of liquid every day. This can be plain spring water, fruit juice diluted 50:50 with water, or any of the beverages mentioned above.

Days Nine and Ten

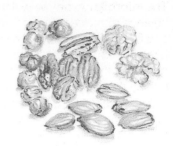

As you near the end of the Ten-day Dietary Detox Programme, begin to increase the variety of foods, especially
proteins. This is a necessary bridge to the more normal
Maintenance regime and the everyday activities that were
put to one side during this intensive detoxification. Remember, now, as always, to chew thoroughly, eat slowly, and so
derive maximum nutritional value from your food. Chewing
well also gives you a truer sense of the point at which you
have eaten sufficiently (known as satiety); this does not
happen when you bolt your food.

● Menu

For breakfast choose *either*:
* Home-made muesli, which should
  include one or two dessertspoons each
  of rolled oats, sunflower seeds, sesame
  seeds, seedless raisins or chopped
  dried fruit, and linseed (flaxseed). Soak
  the ingredients overnight in water and,
  before eating, add a dessertspoon of
  wheatgerm and a finely grated apple, or
  a sliced banana, or sliced papaya. *Or*
* Equal quantities of millet and buckwheat (one to two dessertspoons of
  each) plus a dessertspoonful of linseed
  either soaked overnight in water or
  milled in a processor or nut mill. Plus
  fresh fruit from the list on p.77. *Or*
* Grind in a processor or nut mill a dessertspoonful each of a least four of the
  following: wheat, barley, brown rice,
  oats, rye, linseed, sunflower or pumpkin
  seeds, sesame seeds, and then cook
  approximately three ounces of the resulting mixture in about two cups of
  water until it thickens. Eat this warm
  with additional fruit.

and eat any of the above with:
* Four to eight ounces of live yoghurt and
  additional fresh fruit, if desired.

For lunch or evening meal:
At one of these meals continue to have a
mixed raw salad or lightly-cooked vegetables (steamed or stir-fried), plus either

jacket potato, rice, or banana (but see p.77).
In addition, you may have one or two slices
of wholemeal or rye bread and a little
butter. Have fresh fruit for dessert.

For the other main meal choose from:
* Three ounces (at least) of fish (grilled,
  steamed, or baked but NOT fried). *Or*
* Five ounces (at least) of vegetarian
  savoury (this calls for a mixture of
  grains, pulses, or seeds, see p.85). *Or*
* A plain omelette (two-egg) or boiled or
  poached eggs. *Or*
* Three ounces of chicken (not skin). *Or*
* Fish, chicken, or vegetarian soup (such
  as lentil or bean in the correct combinations as described on p.85).

Eat the above with a variety of mixed vegetables, either steamed, stir-fried, lightly-
boiled, or oven-roasted in olive oil. Dress
cooked vegetables with olive oil and lemon
juice for extra taste.

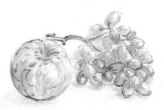

For dessert:
Choose either lightly-stewed fruit, with a
minimal amount of honey for sweetening,
or a baked apple, or fresh fruit.

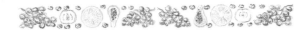

● Balancing foods

The information below will help you understand what balance of nutrients your body needs for optimum health and function. In order to maintain the detoxification process, it is not enough just to provide your body with the raw materials it needs to build healthy tissues; you have to supply them in a balanced manner.

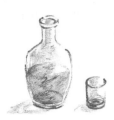

Also refer to p.132-3 to see how some foods can clash during digestion, and how to combine them to avoid this. Read p.136 on how to rotate foods to avoid provoking sensitive and allergic reactions.

● Fat

This should be between 25 and 30 percent of your daily calorie intake, not the 40 percent commoner in the west. Following the menu on p.133) will improve this balance for you. Fish and game are more suitable than domesticated meat such as beef, or pork.

● Carbohydrate

Complex carbohydrates (found in whole grains, pulses, and in all vegetables and fruits) are the basis of good healthy eating. They are also an abundant source of minerals, vitamins, enzymes, as well as other nutrients, (though most people nowadays need to take supplements of these nutrients). Refined carbohydrates (white flour and sugar) are undesirable, though, if the diet is essentially sound, a small amount will do little harm.

● Protein

You can obtain this both from animal and vegetable sources. Fish, game and poultry are the best sources of animal protein: you need to eat between two and eight ounces daily. Vegetarians need roughly double these amounts to ensure balance, and must select the ingredients correctly to get the full spectrum of amino acids (see p.85).

● Raw versus cooked

Ideally at least half your food should be eaten raw. Eat fresh fruit and salad every day and have a side salad with cooked meals. Use fresh fruit rather than cooked for dessert. See p.133 – it's easier than you think.

Appraisal

The Ten-day dietary detox period is nearly over and you should, by now, have noticed some real improvements in your overall health. It is now time to pick up on the dietary pattern in the Maintenance section (p.131). Continue to do relaxation and aerobics at the Basic level for another ten days and gradually incorporate the more advanced Maintenance versions into your life routine. Use the Maintenance section as a guide to teach yourself how to eat and live in a way that will preserve your newfound health.

Every six months, go back to the questionnaires and rescore. The results may indicate that you should start on a dietary detox programme again. If this is the case you can either repeat the Ten-day programme, or follow the slower Thirty-day programme instead. Continue with the exercises and other techniques you have been practising in Maintenance, however, throughout either intensive detox period.

Thirty-day dietary detoxification programme

If you have decided to detoxify more gently than would be the case with the Ten-day programme, for whatever reason (perhaps in order to continue working rather than taking a break at home for an intensive detox), and if your score in the questionnaires indicates that this is appropriate (see p.56 for guidance), then the Thirty-day programme is ideal for you. Throughout the first three weeks of this programme you should practise all the Basic methods which help detoxification, including massage, relaxation methods, hydrotherapy, stretching and aerobic exercises. Towards the end of the programme the more advanced methods described in the Maintenance section should be introduced as and when appropriate.

Weekend One
Start with a two-day intensive detox, using either a fast or a mono-diet (see p.82-3). Start doing the exercises in the Basic programme, and any detox techniques that are not too strenuous. Rest as much as you can. Treat any detox symptoms that appear with the methods on p.60-1. Don't drive while on this strict regime.

Weekend Five
This is your last weekend on the Thirty-day programme. Use it to make one final effort to clear your system through fasting or a mono-diet (p.82-3). Use hydrotherapy and massage to help in this task, and review just how you are going to handle the freedom from the constraints of the programme in your first week on Maintenance. Rescore your questionnaire answers and see how well you have done. Read the notes on the Ten-day programme and see if this would be a better method for you next time.

Week Four
In all essentials this is the same as Week Three. Experiment with the advanced hydrotherapy methods in Maintenance (p.159-65) and use muscle energy-stretching (p.156-7) on any tight areas of your body. Resist the temptation to overdo things; this is a time for reviewing stress and your coping abilities (read p.100 on stress).

Lymphatic massage
This is described on p.170. Use this method whenever you are in the midst of intensive detoxification, since it is when the most active elimination of wastes is underway that the lymph channels (p.179-80) can become overloaded. Massage helps to move the lymph along. Even when there is no one to help you with this specialized massage, do as much as you can by yourself.

Weekend Four
Follow the same dietary pattern as on Weekend Three. There should now be fewer side-effects. Have a massage daily and an Epsom salt bath or a body pack (pp.67 and 165-7) to stimulate elimination through the skin. Practise relaxation, meditation, and visualization at least once every day. Don't drive!

Week One
The crux of the Thirty-day diet is to find a balance between enough food to allow you to work efficiently and yet also allow the process of detoxification to continue. Follow the diet on p.84-5 and continue to use the various components, including all the exercise variations, outlined in the Basic programme (p.62-70).

Weekend Two
On the evening before the second weekend have a light (fruit or salad) meal and try either of the weekend patterns described on p.82-3. Continue with all the elements of the Basic programme and rest as much as possible. Be sure to have a reasonable evening meal on the Sunday night.

Week Two
Follow the same pattern as in Week One. By now you should be feeling benefits from the programme in terms of more energy and a clearer head. If there are signs of skin irritation or nausea apply the methods on p.60-1. Daily bowel movements should be regular, but if not use an enema (p.182) or herbal laxative (psyllium seeds).

Weekend Three
Continue with whichever variation of the rapid detoxification diets suits you best. You can now begin to try more advanced massage, including lymphatic drainage (p.179-80), and the meditation methods outlined on pp.102-3 and 107-10. Mental harmony balances the detoxification of the body. Remember, no driving at weekends.

Week Three
Your midweek detoxification routine should now be well established. Have a massage (p.172) on alternate days, including lymphatic drainage (p.179-80), if needed. Use an appropriate hydrotherapy method several days a week and incorporate meditation and autogenic training (see p.102) in your exercise routines. Your energy levels are now likely to be higher and minor symptoms to have disappeared.

CAUTION: avoid doing anything strenuous during the weekends of the Thirty-day programme, and above all *do not drive*. This is a time for rest, so energy can be diverted to the cleansing and regenerative functions your bodymind now needs.

Choices and results

For your intensive, weekend, detox diet choose between either a one-day fast followed by a day on raw food, or two days on a monodiet (see opposite). Remember that even a short fast or monodiet may produce symptoms of detoxification (as described on p.60 and 141).

● Saturday

For your one-day, water-only fast, prepare to rest and keep warm; you will feel colder than usual. The first experience of detoxification through fasting, with its muzzy head and furred tongue, requires you to be resolute in your determination to continue. As you become less toxic, these symptoms become less obvious (read p.141). Don't give up at the first obstacle: these unpleasant effects are nothing more than evidence of detoxification in action, a process that will later bring you great benefits.

Because you have chosen the slower-acting Thirty-day Dietary Detox Programme it is important to use weekends to full advantage. The fast is the first step. Drink no less than four and not more than eight pints of water through the day. You can freshen its taste with a squeeze of lemon juice if you wish. Always use bottled spring or well-filtered water (see p.116-17).

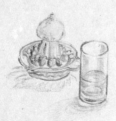

Try to sip the water rather than taking large gulps, and drink some little and often, or whenever you are thirsty or want to freshen your mouth.

● Sunday

On the second day choose between either a raw-food day or a lightly-cooked fruit and vegetable day.

If your choice is raw food, have a fruit breakfast, such as papaya, apple and grapes. Eat each mouthful slowly, chewing exceptionally thoroughly. For lunch and the evening meal have either another fruit meal or a selection of raw vegetables (but without the carbohydrate allowed with the salad meal on the Ten-day programme on p.77). Select your salad so that at least one, and ideally two items are from the range of red/orange vegetables (carrots, beetroot, red cabbage, red pepper, or tomato) and the rest from the vast range of nourishing green salad vegetables and herbs available.

If you have a sensitive digestion (and only if this is so) have cooked fruit and vegetables instead of raw. Fruit can baked or lightly stewed in its own juice or with a little water; the vegetables (the same ones as for the salad meal) can be stir-fried or steamed (see p.134).

On this day drink at least two but not more than four pints of water or potassium broth (see recipe p.76).

Recipe for baked apple or pear
First pierce the skin of the fruit in several places to avoid its exploding in the oven. Then place it in an oven container and cook at baking heat. When the skin looks discoloured (brown or gold) remove it from the oven, open it and pour a little lemon and/or fresh apple juice over it. Let it cool: eat it slowly.

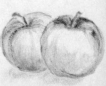

Monodiet

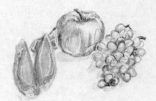

This choice restricts you to eating one food only for two consecutive days (see p.137). This gives your body a chance for detoxification that is just as powerful as fasting and raw days. Read p.141 for advice on dealing with any symptoms that may arise.

Alternatives   Choose *either*

Raw-fruit monodiet: you can eat up to three pounds of your chosen fruit per day (Candida sufferers should first read the note below). *Or*

Cooked-food monodiet: you can eat up to *either* one pound dry weight per day of the grain of your choice, *or* two to three pounds of potatoes.

These foods should be cooked by boiling in water, without using salt; use a little potassium chloride (a salt substitute available from pharmacies or health stores) instead. In addition drink as much plain spring water as you wish.

Eat slowly and chew very thoroughly. Monodiets of the cooked foods listed here are especially useful for people with high blood pressure and high cholesterol levels. They can be eaten cold or warm.

Among the most popular and effective monodiets are:

Raw fruit
* Grapes (preferably eaten with skin)
* Apples (preferably eaten with skin)
* Pears (especially effective if any allergy history)
* Papaya (especially if digestion is sensitive)

Or cooked food (boiled and eaten whenever desired)
* brown rice
* buckwheat
* millet
* potatoes (boiled in their well-washed skins)

One method of making rice (or other foods) more palatable and interesting is to add olive oil and lemon.

Wash rice well, put it in a saucepan, cover it with water; bring it to the boil and simmer until soft (all water should be absorbed). When it has cooled down, add to each serving (one pound dry weight should be adequate for five to six servings when cooked), one half dessert spoonful of olive oil and the juice of one lemon.

Cooked rice without some such addition is difficult to eat. You can treat buckwheat, millet or potatoes in a similar way.

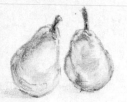
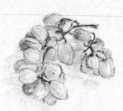

NOTE: during the period of monodieting take daily: one high-potency multi-mineral and one high potency multivitamin tablet/capsule.

CAUTION: anyone with active Candida overgrowth (see p.52) should avoid the fruit monodiet choices, at least until the Candida is under control.

Weekday menus

For breakfast choose from:
*   Home-made muesli, made up from one or two dessertspoons each of: rolled oats, sunflower seeds, sesame seeds, raisins or chopped dried fruit, and linseed (flaxseed). Soak these ingredients overnight in water and, before eating, add a dessertspoon of wheatgerm and some fresh fruit. Eat with four to eight ounces of live yoghurt.
*   Millet and buckwheat (one to two dessertspoons of each) plus a dessertspoon of linseed. Either soak these overnight or grind them in processor or nut mill. Eat with four to eight ounces of live yoghurt and some fresh fruit.
*   A mixture of at least four of the following ground in a processor or nut mill: wheat, barley, brown rice, oats, rye, linseed, sunflower or pumpkin seeds, sesame seeds. Cook approximately three ounces of the resulting mixture in two cups of water until it thickens. Eat warm with live yoghurt and fresh fruit.
*   An all-fruit breakfast and live yoghurt.

Drink herbal tea or lemon and hot water with half a teaspoon of honey.

For lunch choose *either*:
*   Large mixed salad with jacket potato or boiled brown rice (dressed with olive oil, not butter) and either three to four ounces of tofu (bean curd), cottage cheese, or low-fat cheese, or nuts and seeds. *Or*
*   Stir-fried or steamed vegetables eaten with jacket potato or rice, and either cottage cheese, or low-fat cheese, or nuts and seeds.

For supper:
Rotate cooked and raw vegetables between lunch and supper. If you had a cooked-vegetable lunch, have a salad for supper; but if you had a salad lunch you can now have cooked vegetables. If you prefer to have raw salad for both meals, however, do not hesitate to do so.

To accompany the vegetables you can have tofu, cheese, or nuts and seeds as in the lunch menu again. *On alternate days*, however, rotate the cheese accompaniments with either three or four ounces of fish, game, or chicken. This can be either grilled, steamed, boiled, or baked. If you are a vegetarian have a pulse/grain combination that provides a balanced source of protein (see p. 85 for details).

For dessert:
Fresh or lightly stewed fruit (add apple or lemon juice, not sugar, for flavour and sweetness) or natural, live yoghurt.

Supplements
During the entire Thirty-day Dietary Detox Programme continue taking daily one high-potency multivitamin and one high-potency multimineral supplement tablet/capsule. Vegetarians should, in addition, take 15g daily of full- spectrum free-form amino acid tablet/capsules, with water, between meals.

Herbal teas
Some herbal teas are safer than others. Some contain as much tannin as regular tea. The best are linden blossom, chamomile, lemon verbena, sage, and mint. Always drink these between meals, so as to avoid interfering with digestion.

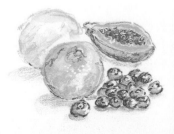

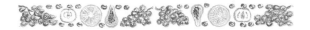

● Vegetarians and protein

The eight amino-acids which are not naturally produced in the body need to be obtained daily from the diet in order to produce the body proteins which are responsible for growth and tissue replacement and the building of functional molecules.

These essential amino-acids need to be present simultaneously and in the right proportions to be usable for protein synthesis. If some are missing, or lacking, some of those present will be "wasted", or used for other purposes such as supplying energy instead, thus creating a need for higher consumption of them to avert the dangers of deficiency.

Animal proteins are highly usable, with milk, cheese and fish ranking even above meat, while soya beans and whole rice are not far behind. Nuts and pulses are only 40–60 percent usable so, because of "wastage", it would be necessary to eat a lot of them to satisfy minimum amino-acid requirements.

For vegetarians the trick is to eat proteins that have mutually complementary amino-acid patterns in such a way that the whole protein value of the meal is greater than the sum of its parts. The most effective combinations from vegetable sources are:

Pulses and grains, e.g. beans on toast, or rice and lentils;

Pulses and nuts and seeds.

How much protein your body needs differs from everyone else's and depends, among other things, on energy output. Department of Health figures recommend a daily minimum of two ounces (55 grams) for a moderately active woman in the 35–65 age range and three ounces (85g) for a similar man. The figure may seem low, but remember it may be necessary to eat far more than these amounts of protein foods to get the recommended amount of pure protein, not all of which is then usable. Whereas fish and meat eaters can get their daily protein from four ounces (115g) of fish or meat, the vegetarian will need eight ounces (225g) of a pulse/grain dish. This is why the additional amino-acid supplement is suggested (opposite) during this period of detoxification, with its restricted eating, and why yoghurt and cottage cheese are such good insurance against protein deficiency.

○ *Rescore*

After you have completed the Thirty-day Dietary Detox Programme, rescore to see what changes have taken place, and then move on to the Maintenance section (p.131). Read through the Ten-day Dietary Detox Programme pages to see whether on another occasion you might like to apply that quicker and more intensive detoxification method instead.

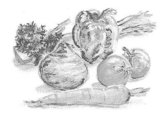

Do
Eat regularly
Chew slowly
Drink at least two pints
of liquid daily
Take multi-vitamin supplements regularly

Don't
Skip meals
Rush your meals
Drink with meals
Eat between meals

Modified programme

This is the place to start detoxification if your score in the questionnaires exceeds 135. Throughout a four week period, follow the diet on p.88-92. This provides for a strict regime at week-ends but a more relaxed though still cleansing pattern midweek. Accompany the diet with complementary exercises and techniques to aid detoxification, starting with the Basic Programme on p.62-73. As you progress with these, you will start introducing the more advanced bodywork techniques in Maintenance.

When you have completed the four weeks, your revised score will guide you to the next step. Whatever dietary advice you are given, however, continue with the bodywork techniques in Maintenance (p.149-57).

Week Four
Stick with the diet you have followed so far, but expand the supportive facets of detoxification as described in the Maintenance section (p.149-81). Rescore your answers to the questionnaires during the week. If your total is now below 135, the next step is to start either the Ten- or Thirty-day Dietary Detox Programmes. If still above 135, you should repeat the Modified Programme.

Pregnancy
Nothing in the Modified Dietary Detox Programme is contraindicated for pregnant women in general. However, if your score in the questionnaires was high enough for you to be referred to the Modified Programme, your level of health is probably poor. You may have special medical problems which need attention, so you should consult your doctor before starting on a detoxification programme.

Weekend Four
This weekend is your last chance to make an intensive effort to clear your system. This oasis of detoxification should be exploited to the full. Make the dietary restrictions as tight as you can, based on the raw food principle (p.79). Use hydrotherapy as strongly as you can and have lymphatic drainage daily. Practice the deeper relaxation methods twice daily and begin to use visualization methods (p.110-11) to bring inner calm.

Week Three
Continue with the deeper relaxation methods (p.107-9) on a daily basis and now incorporate lymphatic-drainage massage (p.170) into your massage sequence. Have this at least every other day from now to the end of the programme. The diet stays the same. You will, by now, be feeling a degree of improvement in your general health. Keep up the effort: you are on the home stretch.

Weekend One

Follow the diet choices given on p.88-9: the aim is at least 60 percent raw food. Start using the body-work methods in the Basic Programme. Take additional supplements of vitamin C and Cysteine (see p.89) as well as the "insurance" multivitamin and multimineral supplements. You may experience slight detox side effects so read p.60-1 for advice.

Week One

Whether you carry out the Modified Programme at home or continue to work, include all facets of detox in your daily routine. The diet described on p.90-2 is not complicated, and allows a gentle degree of detoxification to continue through the week. Do not neglect the Basic Programme methods, however, as they enhance the detox effect. Continue to take the diet supplements suggested on p.89.

Weekend Two

This should, in all essentials, be the same as Weekend One. Use the free time of the weekend intensively for hydrotherapy methods, such as full trunk packs or Epsom salt baths (p.166). Have a massage on each day; continue with the exercises in the Basic Programme. The worst detox side effects will probably occur on this weekend so read p.60-1 again carefully and have first-aid measures (e.g. coffee enema) available when they are needed. Things should start to get better from now on.

Week Two

Follow the same dietary and exercise pattern as in Week One, but expand some of the methods you are using in relaxation and massage. Do not overdo things. Sleep and rest as much as you can without neglecting to use the supportive elements (hydrotherapy and exercise) of the Basic Programme. Read through p.103-11 for guidance on what is to come.

Weekend Three

Intensify detoxification by using either an Epsom salt bath, trunk pack, or peat bath every day. Expand on your relaxation pattern by incorporating autogenic training (p.102) and deeper meditation methods(p.107). Read about these carefully before you start and practise them daily. If you feel a need for general support, adaptogens (p.145) might be appropriate.

Weekend Menus

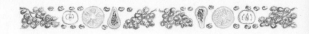

The Modified Dietary Detox Programme is for people with a high initial level of toxicity, and who need to detoxify slowly. It does not include fasts or monodiets, but is aimed at establishing a mainly raw-food pattern. If this presents you with digestive problems, switch to eating lightly-cooked (steamed or stir-fried) food instead. If you start having unpleasant symptoms, read pp.60 and 141-2 for a description of common detox side-effects and their significance. Read p.60-1 for safe treatments.

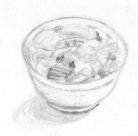

● Menu

For breakfast choose *either*:
* One of the three recipes on p.78 for muesli, seed mixture, or cooked ground grains, plus four to eight ounces of live yoghurt and an item of fresh fruit (papaya would be ideal) or baked or stewed fruit (apple, pear). *Or*
* Oatmeal porridge, eaten with yoghurt rather than milk, with either fresh or lightly-cooked fruit as above.

For lunch eat:
* A mixed raw salad as main course. The selection of salad vegetables should include both green and yellow/orange varieties (e.g. carrot, beet, pepper, cabbage, squash, tomato). *And*
* A baked jacket potato or brown rice (cooked with onion or garlic for more flavour). *And also*
* Two to three ounces of cottage cheese or low-fat cheese.
NOTE: If you have a sensitive digestion and cannot make raw salad a main meal, eat lightly-cooked vegetables (steamed or stir-fried as on p.134) instead. Choose your vegetables as for the salad above, but also eat a small side-salad in addition.

For supper choose from:
* A cooked vegetable mixture (either boiled, baked, steamed, or stir-fried but NOT deep-fried) with one of the following: a one-egg omelette, fish, game, poultry (without skin) or vegetarian savoury. Eat these with a side-salad. *Or*
* A fish, poultry, or vegetarian soup. The vegetarian soup should contain some high-protein foods, such as lentils. Eat these with some wholemeal or rye bread (or toast) and a side-salad.

For dessert have *either*:
* Baked or lightly-stewed apples or pears,
* Fresh papaya. *Or*
* Live natural yoghurt.

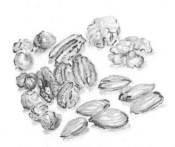

CAUTION: if you are hypoglycaemic (see p.52) eat five small meals each day rather than three large ones.
  If you are pregnant (or have diabetes), check with your doctor before starting on any detoxification programme. Detoxification before conception would be the ideal.

Supplements
Take one high-potency multimineral tablet capsule daily; one high-potency multivitamin tablet/capsule daily; one to two grams of vitamin C in divided doses with meals; and one gram of the amino acid L-cysteine with water at least one hour before or an hour and a half after every meal.

● Special note for allergy sufferers

As you move carefully towards structuring your dietary programme, it is as well to take special note of some allergy facts which may apply to your particular make-up.

If you are allergic to specific foods it is important that you take care to avoid or "rotate" (i.e. eating these no more than once in five days) other foods in the same biological "family" as that food (see p.136). For example, allergy to potato, a member of the Nightshade Family (Solanaceae), could mean that you are also sensitive to tomatoes, peppers or paprika, which are also members of that family.

Allergy to any one of the following members of the Rose Family (Rosaceae) may mean allergy to the others: almond, apple, apricot, cherry, nectarine, peach, pear, plum, rose hip, quince, sloe.

Many of these fruits contain salicylates, a major ingredient of aspirin, to which a large number of people are sensitive or allergic or to which some people suffer a toxicity response. Salicylate sensitivity has been linked to hyperactivity in some children. Be suspicious of these foods if you have ever suffered a bad response to aspirin: almonds, apples, apricots, blackberries, cherries, cucumber, currants, gooseberries, grapes, oranges, peaches, plums, prunes, raisins, raspberries, strawberries and tomatoes. Traces are also found in banana, coffee, pineapple and potato.

Other common allergies occur in the following families:

– Umbelliferae: angelica, caraway, carrot, celery, chervil, coriander, cumin, dill, fennel, parsley and parsnip.

– Compositae: artichoke, chamomile, chicory, dandelion, endive, lettuce, safflower, salsify, sunflower and tarragon.

– Gourd Family (Cucurbitaceae): courgette, cucumber, gherkin, melon, pumpkin, squash, watermelon.

– Grass Family (Graminae): bamboo shoots, barley, bulghur, corn, millet, oat, rice, rye, sorghum, sugar(cane), wheat.

– Laurel Family (Lauraceae): avocado, bay leaf, cinnamon, sassafras.

– Lily Family (Liliaceae): asparagus, chive, garlic, leek, onion, shallot.

– Cabbage Family (Cruciferae), Brassica Tribe: broccoli, brussel sprouts, cabbage, cauliflower, chinese leaves, cress, horseradish, kale, kohlrabi, mustard, radish, turnip, watercress.

If you are sensitive to cow's milk, perhaps the commonest – along with those to the Grass Family (wheat) – of all allergies, then you are probably also reactive to beef, but have a 50 percent chance of being able to tolerate goat's or sheep's milk.

Another common allergy is to gluten, or to wheat which contains gluten. Gluten is a complex of proteins which occurs in wheat and rye and which causes a true toxic reaction in some people, resulting in severe bowel dysfunction (coeliac disease).

This is not at all the same thing as wheat intolerance. People who are allergic to this family of foods suffer true imunological, rather than toxic, reactions. The fact that a food is gluten free does not guarantee that it is wheat free, as gluten can be removed from wheat leaving the wheat allergen still present.

Most people who are wheat sensitive will also react allergically to gluten, but people who are only gluten sensitive do not usually react to wheat once the gluten has been removed.

If you read labels very carefully you may find products which are both gluten and wheat free. Anything containing monosodium glutamate (MSG) is undesirable for a gluten or wheat sensitive individual. And beware: many apparently "safe" flours, such as rice flour, may have added wheat.

Weekday menus

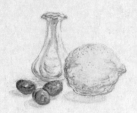

The Modified Dietary Programme is not a difficult one to follow, for it allows far more freedom of choice than the more intensive Ten- and Thirty-day Programmes. It is, in fact, close to the pattern suggested for Maintenance, a life-plan for everyone. Try to avoid slipping into old patterns of eating. Stay within the guidelines as far as is possible, and the benefits will start to flow.

● **Menu One**

For breakfast have:
* Home-made muesli or milled-seed mix (see p.78) and eat it with four to eight ounces of live yoghurt. *And*
* One or two items of fresh or lightly-stewed fruit (see the list on p.77). Use apple juice for sweetening.

For mid-morning drink:
* Herbal tea. *Or*
* Diluted apple juice (50:50 with water), either warm or cold. *Or*
* Lemon juice and hot water with half a teaspoon of honey.

For lunch or supper have *either*:
* A large, mixed salad with a jacket potato or boiled brown rice (dressed with olive oil rather than butter) and three to four ounces of either tofu (bean curd), cottage cheese, or nuts and seeds. If your digestion is sensitive to raw food have the same savoury but eat the vegetables either stir-fried or steamed and dressed in olive oil and lemon juice. *Or*
* A cooked meal with vegetables that are either boiled, steamed, or stir-fried, and either fish or chicken (grilled, steamed, baked or boiled), or an omelette or a vegetarian savoury.

For dessert have:
* Fresh or lightly-stewed fruit. *Or*
* Natural live yoghurt.

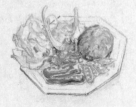

Liquids
During the detoxification period drink not less than two pints of liquid daily in addition to the fluid in the vegetables and salads you are eating anyway.

Choose from bottled spring water, herbal teas (see p.84) or diluted lemon juice (50:50 with spring water, still or sparkling) or lemon juice and hot water plus a quarter teaspoonful of honey or potassium broth (see p.76).

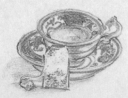

Some recommendations
Particular fruits, such as apples and pears, are less allergenic, as evidenced by clinical experience.

Citrus fruits, though more allergenic, are also recommended, except during fasting when reactions are heightened.

Papaya is one of the easiest of fruits to digest; its seeds, crushed, can be used for tenderizing.

Fresh fruit contains active and beneficial enzymes; these are destroyed by cooking.

Cooking, on the other hand, breaks down the fibrous structures in vegetables, which are otherwise

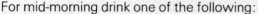

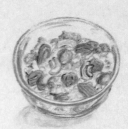

● Menu Two

For breakfast choose:
* Cooked seed-and-grain mix (see p.78) or oatmeal porridge plus four to eight ounces live natural yoghurt. *Or*
* One or two items of fresh or lightly-stewed fruit (papaya, pear, peach, see p.77). Use apple juice for sweetening.

For mid-morning drink one of the following:
* Herbal tea
* Apple juice (diluted) either warm or cold.
* Lemon juice and hot water with half a teaspoon of honey.

For lunch have *either*:
* A large mixed raw salad with jacket potato or boiled brown rice (dressed with olive oil not butter) and three to four ounces of either tofu, cottage cheese, or low-fat cheese, or nuts and seeds. *Or*
* If your digestion is sensitive to raw food, have the same savoury but with lightly-cooked vegetables (steamed or stir-fried) dressed in olive oil and lemon juice. *Or* (best option)

* All fruit, seed (sunflower, pumpkin) and nut (fresh walnuts, almonds, pecans) meal with natural yoghurt.

For supper have:
* A cooked meal of either boiled, steamed, or stir-fried vegetables with a vegetarian savoury combination of pulses (such as lentils, soya protein, tofu, or chickpeas) and grains (whole wheat, brown rice, or millet). *Or,*if you did not have a fruit and nut meal at lunch
* A fruit, nut, and seed meal with yoghurt (see also above).

For dessert have:
* Fresh or lightly-stewed fruit. *Or*
* Natural live yoghurt.

---

hard to digest, and releases the nutrients stored in them.

The reason for selecting live yoghurt is because the useful friendly bacteria, bulgaricus and thermophilus, are killed by the process of sterilization.

The skin of all poultry is very high in saturated fats and is never recommended.

Tap water contains high levels of toxic substances and heavy metals. Spring water is less likely to do so. Glass bottles are purer storage containers than plastic, which may leach.

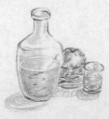

Supplements
Remember to to take the supplements listed on p.89 every day. When you are working a detoxification programme the underlying nutritional support which the multivitamin and multimineral supplement gives is most important. The vitamin C and the L-cysteine provide specific detoxification qualities which greatly assist your body in its cleansing efforts.

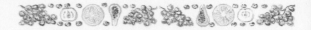

● **Menu Three**

For breakfast:

* All fruit, seed, and nut breakfast with natural yoghurt accompaniment. Eat slowly and enjoy the fresh, rich flavours. Papaya remains the best digested of all fruits and helps with the digestion of others. Yoghurt, if live, also helps digestion and its protein is itself virtually predigested by the friendly bacterial cultures that make it (see p.144)

At mid-morning, drink:

* Herbal tea. *Or*
* Warm or cold diluted apple juice. *Or*
* Lemon juice with hot water and half a teaspoon of honey.

For lunch eat *either:*

* A large, mixed raw salad with jacket potato or boiled brown rice (dress these with olive oil), and three to four ounces of either tofu, cottage cheese, or nuts and seeds. *Or*, if your digestion is sensitive to raw food,

* The same savoury with lightly-cooked vegetables (the same selection as for salad). Either stir-fry or steam these and dress with olive oil and lemon juice rather than butter.

For supper choose from:

* Fish or chicken (without the skin), either boiled, steamed, stir-fried, baked, or grilled with lightly-cooked vegetables, or else the vegetables and an omelette.

Lunch and supper menus can be transposed if you prefer.

For dessert:

* Fresh or cooked fruit. *Or*
* Natural live yoghurt.

○ *Rescore*

When you have completed a month on the Modified Detoxification Programme you should rescore for ALL the questionnaires. If your score is now below 135, you should then embark on either the Ten-day or Thirty-day Dietary Detox Programmes and after that move on to the Maintenance Programme. If your score is still above 135 you should spend another month on the Modified Programme but continuing with the body/mind technique levels of Maintenance (Part 3) as explained on p.56-7.

PART THREE

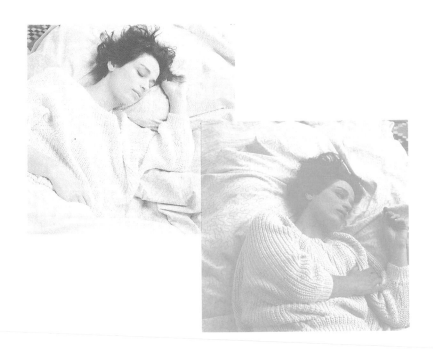

Maintenance

● Introduction

Life is, above all, for living and, important as the periodic intensive detoxification programmes are, they are no substitute for the sort of daily habits that keep you clear, detoxified and vital.

You will derive some benefits if all you do is follow detoxification programmes from time to time, while carrying on with whatever behaviour got you into a toxic state in the first place; but this is a pretty short-sighted approach to life.

The regular servicing of any machine, an automobile for instance, is vital if you want it to perform well. But if you treat it badly between services (drive in the wrong gear perhaps, or, worse still, use the wrong fuel) its useful life will be severely curtailed. Servicing will keep it going longer than if you did nothing at all, but it is the way an automobile is used every day, the way you maintain it, that really decides its life.

The marvellous machine in which you live differs from a machine such as an automobile in this important respect: your body has, inbuilt, the ability to repair itself – if it is given the chance. Detoxification periods are the "service" breaks which give you just such a chance. But it is what you do in between that really decides how well and how long your "machine" will last. This is where your choice of "fuel", and how well or badly you treat yourself, and to what unpleasant and toxic substances you expose yourself, greatly influence just what level of wellbeing you will enjoy.

The life plan which follows is a guide to relatively toxin free living. It includes attention to both mind and body, for mental stress is as toxic as (some say more than) any poison in the air, our water or food.

As you read through these pages, refer back to Part One to remind yourself of just what, and how well-established, the enemy is. The ideas built into the life plan can provide you with a weapon which, effectively wielded, can win for you a high level of health and vitality.

NOTE: Do not start work on Maintenance until you have done the Ten-day or Thirty-day Dietary Detox Programme. Why? Because, quite simply, the various components of the programmes build on each other; you need to do one before you can do another. If you have only gone through the Modified Programme so far, you now need to do either the Ten-day (p.74) or the Thirty-day (p.80) Dietary Detox Programme before starting on Maintenance.

Life plan

The various components of the Maintenance Programme, which you will find in the following chapters, are like parts of a jig-saw puzzle: they fit together to create a "picture of health", but some pieces need to be used more frequently than others. For aerobics to have any real long-term effect, for example, you need to exercise at least three times a week, preceded by warm-up stretching exercises. At least once (ideally twice) a week you should spend time doing a full stretching session using all the Basic and Maintenance positions to loosen and free the body. Once or twice weekly you should also have a fully body massage combined, if possible, with one of the detoxifying hydrotherapy methods. Step hydrotherapy and massage up to once a day in times of extra exposure to toxicity, or if a cold or flu is threatening.

The relaxation breathing which leads on to meditation and then to visualization should be a part of your daily life (many believe that twice a day is the ideal) for not less than 20 minutes. In times of stress this should be increased, either in length of time or number of times practised. Try to follow the general dietary guidelines on p.131–47 and think in terms of periodic detoxification; how often will depend on what time you can spare.

Some people choose to have a two day/weekend fast or monodiet every six weeks or so, as well as a Ten-day or Thirty-day Dietary Detox once a year (after checking the questionnaire score in case the Modified Programme is needed first). This could be seen as the ideal. Other people choose a "raw food" day once a week or fortnight to keep the detox process going, coupled with an annual "spring clean" (the time of year is optional).

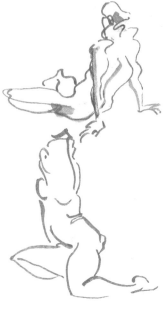

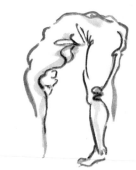

Monday, Wednesday, Friday
Wake 6.30am
20 minutes breathing/relaxation
　meditation
10 minutes yoga stretching
Home from work 6.30pm
5 minutes warm-up exercises
25–30 minutes brisk walk, skipping or cycling
Full body skin friction before bath or shower

Tuesday, Thursday
Wake 6.30am
20 minutes breathing/relaxation/visualization
　10 minutes yoga stretching
An hour and a half after evening meal
Full body relaxation massage, followed by
　Epsom salt bath

Saturday
Wake 8.30am
30 minutes breathing/relaxation/visualization
10 minutes yoga stretching
Later that afternoon or evening
Full body massage or local massage to area in
　need, followed by
Body or trunk pack or sitz bath

Sunday
Wake 8.30am
30 minutes breathing/relaxation/meditation/
　visualization
10 minutes yoga stretching
Mid-morning
5 minutes warm-up exercises
25–30 minutes brisk walk, skipping or cycling

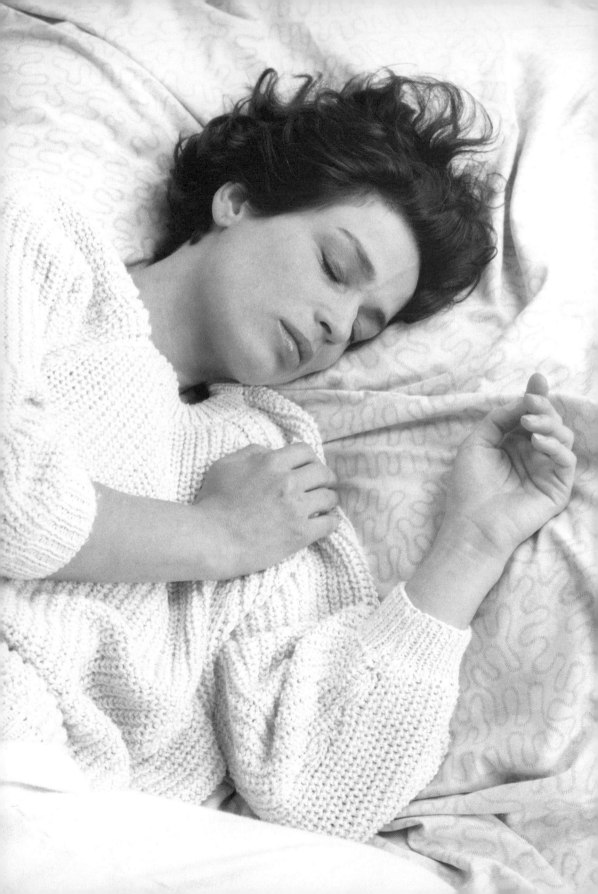

Detoxifying the Mind

A need to detoxify the mind may at first seem surprising, especially when the need to clean up the environment and our physical state are so obvious. However, it is your mind that is the ultimate control system; the functions it performs make it the epicentre of your whole being. And, unfortunately, you have probably allowed this magnificent machine to become toxified through limited beliefs, distorted thinking, negative attitudes and "broken records" – those little voices in the head that chant *can't, should, ought* and *must*.

Added to this, you are, very likely, upsetting the brain's delicate biochemical balance with a whole range of dangerous substances, ingested compliments of our polluted food chain – impurities, additives and toxins – never mind drugs, alcohol and other chemicals.

Disease does not "happen" in isolation. Even a summer cold can be traced to a time of difficulty or high stress. There are reasons for all changes in your body; many of these reasons are in your mind. If you are now striving toward a more harmoniously balanced lifestyle, by lessening the effects of our toxic civilization, then now is the right time for you to rediscover the natural healing power you were born with.

We recognize a difference between the positive person's response to stressful situations and that of others who feel powerless, overwhelmed, or weighted down. The emotionally balanced see problems as challenges to be overcome; they feel in control of the situation, and can utilize the stress factor in a positive way. The others will more easily become ill and have more difficulty in maintaining balance in health, emotions and thinking.

Negative stress reactions, themselves caused by negative emotions, attitudes and addictions, displace the natural healing energy you were born with. Healing begins with detoxifying the mind/brain and effectively utilizing your natural stress reaction. But first we will examine how this equation adds up to a *negative* stress response instead of a *positive* one.

Some attitudes and emotions, such as fear, hatred, jealousy, resentment, desire for revenge or dominance are as destructive as the physical toxins we spend so much time and effort confronting. Indeed, they are self-destructive, since they have specific and far-reaching influences on your health. When they are allowed to die away, they make room for the positive emotions which enhance our recovery and protect our health.

Understanding addiction, altering attitudes, changing self-destructive emotions, understanding reaction, so that the energy stress produces is rechannelled into productive self-healing, is the purpose of this section. It introduces you to more advanced relaxation, meditation and visualization methods, building on the Basic programme you have already started. Applying these techniques releases previously locked-in energies, promotes a sense of both well-being and worth, and allows your mind to act in concert with your body in achieving positive, high-level wellness.

Now re-read the questions on p.45-8, and your answers.

Attitudes and emotions

Attitudes may be described as beliefs formed by parental "programming": they dictate a manner of acting, feeling or thinking that expresses those beliefs. These attitudes are acquired through parents, school, church, friends and relatives throughout life. During childhood we usually accept the attitudes we are given without question. Later on our life experiences teach us more permanent attitudes about "the way things are", no matter how self-destructive. Fortunately, since attitudes are learned, they can be changed. If you have developed negative or self-destructive attitudes you may find it necessary to change them by becoming aware of the attitudes you hold; learning about other ideas and challenging the old ones; asking yourself what attitudes need changing to enhance your recovery; and allowing yourself to have new and positive life experiences which reflect changing attitudes.

As your attitudes change, so will your feelings. Why? Because your thoughts create your emotions, which in turn act as a mirror to expose your thinking. They can either become linked in a vicious cycle leading to depression, dysfunction and serious physical dis-ablement; or you can regain mastery through understanding, and use healthy attitudes to generate positive, healthy feelings.

Although emotions and thoughts are bound up together, trying to talk yourself out of a particular feeling isn't very effective. This is easy to understand if you are unfortunate enough to suffer from a phobia. Phobias are born in the mind, put there by negative experiences, but embedded in the emotions where they grow out of proportion and control, just like cancer. The only way to help someone with a phobic response is to rediscover the initial damaging incident, and this is hard work, even for professionals.

If you have already tried "positive thinking" without success, you may have missed out the most important aspect: using positive thoughts as an overlay to blot out negative feelings is not enough. They leave the original unpleasant feelings generated by the powerful underlying attitudes untouched. Worse, you may now feel a failure, and then guilty for failing. This vicious circle can be broken by seeking to understand your internal thinking process. This leads to changes in attitude and creates a positive upward spiral. It is hard work, but the results are worth it.

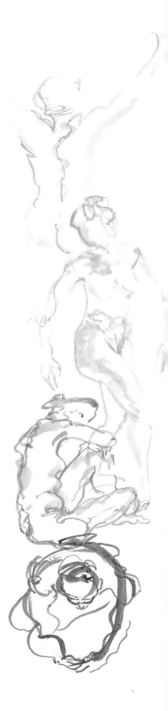

Addiction

Isn't it strange how we have accepted the proposition that the causes of all our difficulties are outside us? Society has taught us that the cure will be found outside, too, in the form of prescriptive drugs, or self-prescribed alcohol, food, sex, or so on. What would happen to your problems and disorders if you began to "take charge" of your life by changing your attitudes, becoming response-able for your emotions, by recovering from ALL your addictions and by utilizing your stress response effectively?

Addiction is a difficult subject which most people would rather not examine. The subject is further complicated because addiction takes so many forms, and even the experts disagree about its causes. It may be described as a physical and/or emotional dependence on a substance or behaviour which becomes the unifying principle around which one's life is lived. In the past, "addiction" meant drugs or alcohol. In reality, millions of people are food addicts, sex addicts, or are addicted to gambling, shoplifting, or they are addictive spenders, or workaholics. Even relationships can be addictive and destructive. The desire to feel better or to alleviate uncomfortable feelings is common to all addictions.

Over time, people suffering with addictions develop an "addictive personality": the thinking, feeling and entire lifestyle of an individual changes in order to hide, protect and sustain the addiction. Fear, disgust, shame and self-hatred are inevitable consequences, causing the addict to use the substance or behaviour to mask these negative feelings. Isolation, loneliness and despair are the companions of those who do not know how to break free of their self-destructive cycles.

Removing the substance or stopping the behaviour is only the beginning. Indeed, it is not enough simply to remove the substance or addictive behaviour, for the addict may just switch to something else. The distorted personality system remains in place as long as ANY addictive behaviour is indulged in. For most people, total abstinence from alcohol, for example, will be a necessary basic requirement for recovery, but recovery means restoring a whole and balanced personality and lifestyle. This includes resocialization, learning about the addiction process, talking about the problems with other recovering addicts, and making basic changes in thinking and feeling. Twelve step support groups such as Alcoholics Anonymous or Narcotics Anonymous can be very helpful with all these aspects of recovery.

If you scored high in the "soft" drug section, you need to examine your reliance on substances to change your moods. They do long-term damage to your adrenal glands. Try carob instead of chocolate; herbal teas, fruit and vegetable juices in place of cola, and decaffeinated drinks.

If you scored high in the use of medicinal drugs, you should consult a qualified medical adviser for guidance. Stopping prescriptive medications on your own can be dangerous.

If your overall score was high in this section (see p.48) start the Modified programme, p.86, but do NOT work the Basic programme until your score drops appropriately.

Stress

Stress is a normal human condition on which we depend for survival. An early example of stress functioning correctly was our ancestors' wise decision to run from sabre-toothed tigers. Functioning incorrectly, however, it wastes energy and threatens our health. Since stress is a natural reaction to situations which require our energy and attention, it can, and even should, be our friend. When we learn to cope with stress, to see change as a challenge not a threat, we reduce damage and can benefit from experiences which would otherwise harm us.

What makes some people more efficient at coping with stress? Perhaps the "hardiness factor", one aspect of which is **commitment**, the ability and willingness to be involved in what is happening around you. The "loner" who withdraws from social contact demonstrates the opposite of this. The second aspect is **control**, characterized by the belief that you can influence events by the way you feel, think, and act. The opposite of this is feeling that events or people control you. The third aspect is **challenge**, in which there is an expectation of change in life and that most changes are welcomed as leading to personal development. The opposite of this is fear and dislike of any sort of change. This negative reaction causes rigidity leading to obsessive/compulsive personality traits.

If you recognize any of these negative elements in yourself, then the energy that stress produces to save you from sabre-toothed tigers, may be causing you harm. Detoxification helps you to use the power of deep relaxation meditation to "stress-proof" yourself. By learning to breathe, meditate, relax your mind and body, you will be able to change your attitudes and finally your behaviour. You will learn to respond instead of react to challenging situations. This is the beginning of self-mastery, a state which may be described as effective utilization of an unlimited energy source.

High-scorers on Stress questionnaire
Practice the sequence of deep breathing, p.63, progressive muscular relaxation p.64, autogenic training, p.102, meditation, p.107, then visualisation, p.110, at least once and ideally twice daily for 20-30 minutes at a time. Also consciously try to use elements of the "hardiness" factor to increase your stress-coping abilities.

When faced with a stressful situation, or when agitated during withdrawal, breathe in through the nose, filling your lungs in 2-3 seconds. Pause for a second, then breathe out to a silent count of 7 or 8 seconds. Repeat till the agitation passes. Breathe normally for a while before resuming activity.

Well-researched scientific experiments have shown this ancient yoga breathing pattern to be effective in "switching off" panic attacks and episodes of hyperventilation.

● **Changing behaviour patterns**
Smoking   Smoking usually involves both a psychological and a physical dependence; both need to be considered as you try to quit. The one vital element in stopping is wanting to: with this motivation it is always possible to do so.

If you intend to continue to smoke, you can slightly protect your body, and the bodies of those living with you,

by means of the healthy diet and supplementary programmes described in this book.

If you intend to stop smoking, the following may help:
*   For the first 4–6 weeks take a high potency vitamin B
    complex tablet, (at least 50mgs each of the major B
    vitamins) daily with food, and also 500 mgs each of the B
    vitamins Niacinamide and Pantothenic acid. They may
    turn your urine dark yellow or green, but this is all right.
*   Acupressure with the thumb nail for up to a minute at a
    time, several times a day, will reduce many withdrawal
    symptoms. Points to press (never use a needle) are
    illustrated on p.73. Use the hand point for headache,
    restlessness, cough and tight chest; the leg point for
    indigestion and nausea, as well as the main "nausea"
    point on the forearm.
*   Relaxation and breathing methods on p.63-5.

Drinking   The more alcohol you drink the more you are
likely to be protein, and therefore amino acid, deficient. So
*   Take a combination of all the amino acids in their "free"
    form (virtually predigested) in doses of between 500 and
    1000 mgs three times daily, with vitamin B6 (100mgs) on
    an empty stomach an hour before meals. Plus 500 – 1000
    mgs of amino-acid L-glutamine three times a day with
    water, away from meals. This combination both reduces
    craving and enhances nutritional status dramatically.
*   Use the same acupressure points as indicated for smok-
    ing to help reduce withdrawal symptoms.
*   Meditation, p.107, will help too.

Time   If you scored high on p.44, think how to modify your
time allocation. Unbalanced organization of time may lead to
imbalance in health.

Organise time each day for hobbies, meditation, exercise
and socializing. Make a year-long schedule, with periods of
complete contrast from normal activity. Take periodic weekend breaks as well as longer holidays. And plan on a weekly
basis for outings, hobbies, sport or lazing about.

Above all, ensure enough time for sleep, whether 7 to 8
hours at night, or a shorter night-time sleep plus afternoon
nap. We need to sleep deeply and soundly, to dream and
thus obtain both physical and mental rejuvenation. The
energy released during sleep is employed in essential
maintenance and repair; a good deal of detoxification takes
place during sleep.

Sleeping tablets usually prevent the dream process and
lead to dependency very
rapidly. A combination of 1g
of the amino acid tryptophan
and 50mgs vitamin B6 be-
fore sleep on an empty
stomach, however, is a non-
addictive medication which
does not interfere with
dream cycles (see p.111).

Autogenic training

The sequence of relaxation methods in the programme takes you through breathing retraining, muscular relaxation and on towards meditation. The interface between the purely mental activity of meditation and the obviously physical activity of progressive muscular relaxation is a marvellous area in which you learn to focus your mind on parts of the body in a set pattern. This is called autogenic training (AT), and is itself a form of meditation in that it asks the mind to focus on only one thing at a time.

The version described here modified from the full AT sequence will enhance physical relaxation as well as teach you how to keep your attention focused. This is helpful for the meditation methods which follow on p.107.

The mechanics of AT call for you to take up a suitable reclining position, preferably more than an hour after a meal, and certainly not when you are likely to be disturbed or to have to rush off on some activity. Make sure that you are warm and comfortable (no tight clothing, no distracting sounds). After some deep relaxation breathing, focus attention first on your dominant hand or arm. Visualize that arm or hand becoming, or feeling, extremely heavy. Then make a silent statement to yourself, "My arm feels (or is getting) heavy". After this affirmation, spend 10-15 seconds observing the arm, sensing the weight of it, its inertia as it sinks into the floor. Repeat this affirmation once or twice more, always followed by a period of observation, focusing, and sensing.

If you find it helpful, record the text opposite, or a modification of it, so that your own voice provides the affirmations at appropriate intervals.

Gradually pass around the body – to the other arm, one leg and then the other, before returning to the dominant arm to start a new sequence. This time use the affirmation, "My arm is feeling (getting) warm". The exact same sequence is then followed around the body. Finally pay attention to your forehead and make the mental statement that "It feels cool". After a minute or so say to yourself, "I feel refreshed and relaxed". Stretch, sit up, make sure you are not dizzy and continue your day with new energy.

Whether or not you sense the heaviness, you are certainly learning to stay with your attention in one place. Initially there will be a tendency to wander into other thought patterns. When this happens, gently return the mind to its focal point – the arm or hand.

If at any time you really feel the sense of warmth or

How often?
To start with, do this exercise every other day, alternating with progressive muscular relaxation, p.64, but in any case always preceded by a relaxation breathing sequence, p.63. After some weeks, stop progressive muscular relaxation and do AT daily.

heaviness, stay with it, let it spread, sense the deep relaxation it carries with it. It is interesting to note that a skin thermometer attached to a limb in which this is being done will show a rise in temperature as the muscles relax and allow a better circulatory flow.

Timing varies, but as a rule stay for about a minute on each of the four main points of focus – arms and legs – with each of the affirmations – heavy and warm – as well as the final minute on the forehead focus. Combined with the preliminary breathing, this exercise adds up to a minimum of ten minutes.

NOTE: You should not start this exercise until you have already spent some weeks practising the breathing pattern outlined on p.63, and the progressive relaxation exercise on p.64.

○ *Text for taping*
"My right arm (hand) feels (is getting) heavy". Pause for 15 seconds while you sense this. Repeat once or twice more.

"My left arm feels heavy". Pause. Repeat.
"My left leg feels heavy". Pause. Repeat.
"My right leg feels heavy". Pause. Repeat.
"My right arm (hand) feels (is getting) warm(er)".
Pause, sense tingling warmth. Repeat phrase and pause once or twice.

"My left arm feels warm". Pause. Repeat.
"My left leg feels warm". Pause. Repeat.
"My right leg feels warm". Pause. Repeat.
"My forehead feels cool". Pause. Repeat.

Put a small pillow under your head and something to support your knees in a flexed position, to ease any strain on the lower back while doing this exercise.

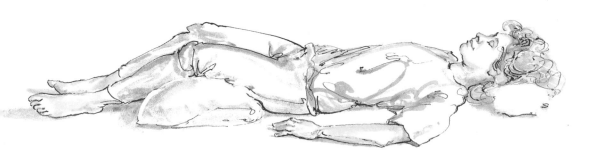

Muscle energy methods

Muscles use more energy than any other part of the body. Most of the time we tend to hold them in a state of greater tension than is actually necessary. This wastes a great deal of energy, and eventually makes them less elastic and more fibrous. Muscles that are constantly tense also seriously slow down the efficient drainage of wastes from tissues through the lymphatic and normal circulation channels. Release of unnecessary tensions is therefore important for more than just energy-saving reasons. We can release some tension through exercise, relaxation exercises, massage and stretching as part of our detox programme.

Whether tensions in muscles are the result of emotional states (anger and fear, for example, dramatically increase muscle tone) or of postural or other tensions, you can learn to release and relax them effectively and painlessly. We know that unless muscular tensions are relaxed, the mind cannot be really calm. When we find ways of achieving muscular release, the mind can be taken to its quietest state in the meditation that follows.

Osteopathic medicine has devised a simple method of releasing tight muscles through isometric contractions. An isometric contraction takes place when a muscle is prevented from moving while contracted. The neurological effect of holding such a muscle thus for 7-10 seconds is to enable the muscle to relax more than it could before, and stretch out to a more normal length. This physiological principle is called post-isometric relaxation – PIR for short.

A second principle derives from the fact that all muscles have "antagonists" which perform the function opposite to their own. Thus, after an isometric contraction, the muscle opposing the contracting muscle will be forced to relax too due to "reciprocal inhibition", RI for short, and it too can be stretched more easily than before.

After an isometric contraction, take the muscle to its new resting length without forcing it, without any pain, and then repeat the contraction, using either the tight muscle itself or its antagonist to produce relaxation, and before stretching it a little more afterwards.

Use this technique to release tight muscles which fail to relax in spite of progressive muscular relaxation, p.64, or autogenic training methods, p.102.

If the main muscle of the upper arm (biceps) is tight, place your other hand on the forearm and resist an attempt to bend it; an isometric contraction will result. After ten seconds of mild effort applied in this way, the muscle will relax and allow itself to be more easily stretched out. Alternatively, if resistance is applied to the other side of the forearm, and the arm resisted as it tries to straighten, then the antagonist muscle (triceps) will be affected.

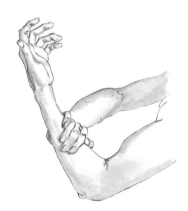

CAUTION: never use more than gentle amounts of strength (say 20% of that available) when you make these contractions, and do not use them in parts of the body where you have joint problems, such as an arthritic neck, without first discussing this with your medical adviser.

This sequence of neck stretching exercises helps to improve the balance of muscle tone in the neck, allowing for greater freedom of drainage of lymph from, and of circulation of blood to and from, the head.

If you have particular neck problems get medical approval of these essentially safe methods before starting. At no time use more than light muscular effort – say 20% of available strength – and always start and finish both the contraction and the resistance slowly. After the contraction, gently stretch the neck towards the direction you were pushing with the head. Repeat several times until no more improvement is noticed.

For relief of muscular neck stiffness sit on a stool in shower, legs apart, spine bent forward, hands behind neck, elbows pulling lightly towards the floor, while hot water plays on the muscles of the upper back and neck. Add to relaxation and stretching by introducing gentle isometric contractions against the hands with the head and neck, then further stretching.

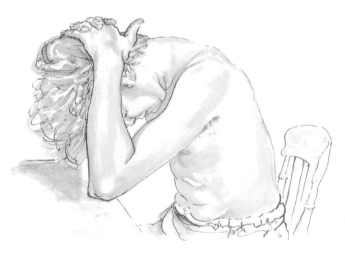

Sit with elbows on table, hands clasped behind head bent forward to comfortable limit. Using light pressure try to take head back and up as hands resist. Hold for ten seconds and slowly release. Then stretch neck into greater forward bending and hold for ten seconds.

With hands supporting forehead, press head forward, tucking chin in to chest, and resist with the hands. Hold for ten seconds and slowly release. Stretch head carefully backwards and hold for several seconds before repeating.

Left hand over top and slightly right of head, resist gentle effort to take head towards right shoulder. Hold for ten seconds, release and stretch head towards left shoulder. Repeat on other side.

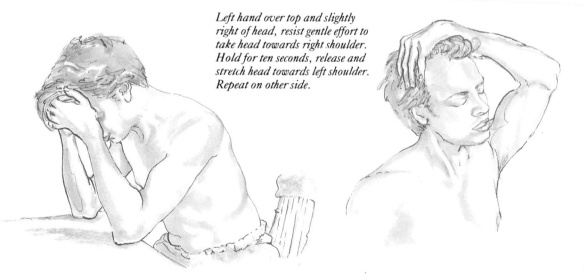

This isometric method allows you to stretch the many small muscles of the spine, freeing much tension, and increasing mobility and suppleness. Instead of applying hand pressure against an effort, as in the neck exercises on the previous page, you will rely on gravity to stretch the muscles. Use this exercise whenever you feel back stiffness, and in any case once or twice a week for general stretching. It is safe if you follow the guidelines carefully.

Lie on your back with your left side near the edge of a bed. Raise right leg and twist lower trunk so leg hangs over the edge, foot dragging towards the floor. Keep left leg straight. Grasp right side of bed with right arm for stability and turn head to the right. This twists the lower half of your body to the left, the upper half to the right.

Raise the right leg a few inches towards the ceiling so that the muscles of the low back tighten slightly.

Hold for ten seconds; slowly release, allowing leg to drag down towards the floor, stretching the back muscles. Stay for 30 seconds, then change round and repeat everything on the other side.

Vary the angle of the leg (point it more or less towards the foot of the bed) to stretch other muscles in the back.

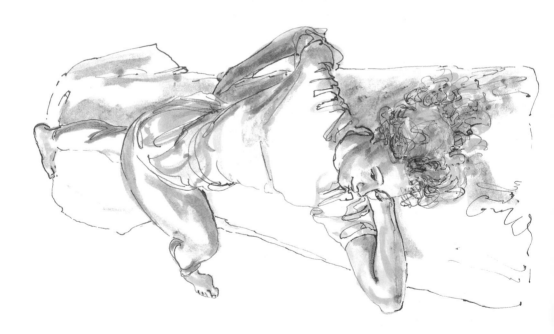

CAUTION: do not attempt this exercise if you have back problems, or have an arthritic condition in the hips, without permission from your doctor.

Meditation

All forms of meditation – and there are many – have in common the attempt to focus the non-critical mind on one object, whether this is a sound, an image, a phrase or word, an idea or an activity. One immediate result of meditation is a change in the pattern of electrical waves in the brain so that an intensely calming sequence of alpha and theta waves develops leading to a state of alert calmness. In consequence a number of profoundly beneficial physiological changes start to take place, not least the reduction of stress and tension, and the disappearance of many stress-related symptoms such as high blood pressure, digestive problems and insomnia.

How Often?
As your practice of meditation becomes established, so you can reduce the amount of time spent on breathing and relaxation exercises, although a few minutes spent on these can lead you gently into meditation each time. Your objective is to meditate daily (twice daily when stress levels are high) for not less than ten and, ideally, twenty minutes at a time.

In addition, it is in this state of calmness that behaviour patterns involving addiction are able to alter, allowing easier withdrawal. Anyone giving up smoking or withdrawing from alcohol or drugs should find meditation a most powerful aid.

Suitable forms of meditation, regularly repeated (daily at least), almost always result in greater mental composure, reduced levels of irritability, enhanced ability to concentrate and a feeling of greater energy. For many people meditation also allows an awakening of spiritual awareness and an expansion of consciousness.

It is not possible to reach a meditative state successfully until you have learned to relax, which is why you have been asked to go through the sequence of breathing exercises, muscular relaxation exercises and autogenic training.

Meditation is a most remarkable way of maintaining a calm and healthy mind in the face of the stresses of modern life. It can be seen as the ultimate mental detoxification tool and its proven enhancement of physical functions makes it essential for all forms of detoxification.

On p.108 five different forms of meditation are described. Try each for some days to see which suits you best, before settling on one for your own personal use. When you first meditate you will find that your mind still wanders, that there is an inevitable "chatter" of thoughts interrupting the stillness you want. Do not worry or become agitated; this is quite normal. Each time, just gently replace the intrusive thoughts with the meditation object, and with time and practice you will develop the ability to stay quietly alert and focused for the entire period of the exercise.

Meditation

Find 20-30 uninterrupted minutes and a quiet room with
comfortable lighting. Choose an object to focus on. Induce
relaxation through deep controlled breathing for a few
minutes; allow the breathing pattern to find its own rhythm.
You will find it helpful to adopt one of the postures illustrated opposite. It may also help if you allow your eyeballs to
roll upwards, eyelids open, until you feel a mild muscular
discomfort. Maintain this for some seconds and then gently
close the eyelids, keeping the eyeballs rolled upwards.
Alternatively, just close your eyes.

Using an Image Focus your mind on an imaginary object
such as a cross, candle flame or circle of light. Concentrate
attention on the object, and as the mind tries to slip away to
other thoughts, gently return to the object of your meditation. With repetition you will learn to stay focused on the
object for 10-20 minutes.

Using sound Introduce a sound into your thoughts. This
sound is not expressed out loud but inside your mind. In the
Eastern tradition this mantra is chosen by a teacher and may
be a sacred word such as "om" or "raam". Research has
shown that any repetitive sound will do; the philosopher
Krishnamurti even suggested that "coca-cola" or "banana"
would work as well as a mystical sound. Allow the repetition
of the chosen sound to blot out thoughts which will continue to try to intrude. Eventually the sound becomes
blurred and ends as a droning blanket throughout the
meditation period. It is the *focusing* on the sound which is of
the essence.

Using a phrase or idea Instead of a repetitive sound,
introduce a repetitive phrase or idea into the mind. This, too,
can be sacred if appropriate to you – "God is love", for
example – or a general idea such as love, truth or peace. The
word, phrase or idea is there to clear the mind of the chatter
of thoughts which are accustomed to circulate there.

Using colour If this is something you are comfortable
with, visualize a stream of coloured light entering or flowing
through your body. First see orange, red or yellow light
slowly flowing, one at a time, upwards into your solar
plexus. Then see a green river of light coming into the same
region from directly in front of you. Spend a minute or two
with each colour. Visualize blue, indigo and violet flowing

down from above and being breathed into you. Finally, see yourself bathed in blue light, and feel the intense calm this produces.

Using touch   In the Middle East worry beads are used to reduce stress. The repetitive movement of the beads around the chain, the feel of the material, and the gentle sound of their movement all induce a meditative state. You can also use a few pebbles: feel their texture, shape and temperature as they move from hand to hand, or as the fingers caress them. Focusing attention on the tactile sensations produced by handling such objects allows the meditation process to arise.

Choose a comfortable position for meditation so your attention can focus on its chosen object without distraction. Sit normally in a chair or try out these variations to see which suits you best. Whichever you choose, keep the spine straight to avoid distracting muscular discomfort.

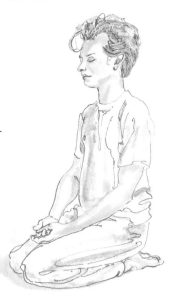

The full lotus position is only suitable for yoga devotees who have stretched the appropriate muscles. The modified position, illustrated here, is comfortable for most people.

Sitting on the heels, with feet pointing backwards, allows the spine to be held tall with consequent opening of the rib-cage – vital for free breathing. The hands rest on the thighs, either with thumb touching index finger as for the lotus, or in quiet repose.

If these two postures are uncomfortable, adopt the yoga "corpse" position. The main disadvantage of this position is the likelihood of your falling asleep – not at all the intention of meditation.

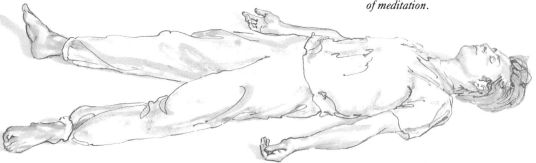

Visualization

The mind can be brought to the support of healing processes in even very serious diseases. One technique for channelling it to this end is visualization. Visualization means "seeing", in whatever terms make sense to you, your body helping to put right whatever is wrong with it. In conditions as diverse as rheumatic pain, cancer, AIDS and acne, varying degrees of benefit have been found to follow persistent visualization or "guided imagery". These methods are now being used more and more extensively as a complementary programme alongside conventional medical methods, at centres as far apart as Harvard Medical School, Mass., and Charing Cross Hospital, London.

Successful visualization is best achieved by people who have mastered the basic essentials of relaxation and meditation; this is why it was necessary for you to practise these first steps for some weeks before proceeding.

● Safe Haven

Follow breathing, relaxation and meditation with the visualization of a safe haven. Spend several minutes seeing yourself in a scene which you find pleasant and safe. It can be real or imaginary, and can vary from time to time in any way you choose. It should contain as many elements as possible which impinge on your senses. So, if you visualize yourself sitting by a river bank, you should not only "see" it but "hear" the ripple of the water and the song of the birds; "smell" the flowers, "feel" the softness of the grass and the brushing of your face with the willow branches and the warmth of the sun on your skin. A total experience will be built up as you exercise the powers of visualization. Do this every time you meditate. Change it, improve it, elaborate on it in any way you wish — it is *your* safe haven.

After you have practised this for some weeks, introduce images of any healing process you think needs reinforcing in you. In detoxification terms you could "see" those parts of you which cleanse and eliminate working superbly efficiently to deal with remaining toxic wastes. You could "see" blemishes heal, and perhaps visualize yourself in a situation in which, when a "tasty toxin" is offered to you, you happily decline. To be successful, images must be positive not negative; try to think, "I am full of energy" rather than, "I am no longer as exhausted as I was".

Dreams
As you begin to go deeper into relaxation, meditation and, eventually, visualization, so your dreams will begin to alter and become more relevant and meaningful. There is much evidence to suggest that dreams are often a sort of coded message from your unconscious mind — virtually a mental detoxification process in themselves, and they may have much to tell us if only we can decipher them.

You may find that some are clear and easy to read while others seem unconnected with your life or problems. An understandable pattern may emerge in time, and dream note books are a great help; however hard you try, you are unlikely to remember your dreams accurately without them.

Visualization
Sit in a comfortable position. Now start to visualize an area in your body where you feel the core of any trouble to be. Allow an image to appear which represents the problem — it may help to paint or draw a symbol or picture. Have the image as clear as possible, including colour, shape, size, even smell. Now feel your body being filled with the power to recreate the picture. Introduce anything you need to make it more healthy, and see the image changing until it is acceptable and in quiet harmony with the rest of your being.

Relax in a comfortable position. Imagine yourself lying on the soft, warm sand of a beautiful beach under a cloudless blue sky. Relax your body until you feel yourself melting into the sand, its grains shifting to accommodate your shape and its firmness supporting you perfectly. Allow every part of your body to let go of any tension, and then become aware of each breath becoming even and deep. Now look up at the sky and imagine a symbol or word, representing any current problem, blazoned above in white, like the vapour trail of an aeroplane. As you watch, the trail fades gradually into insignificance, allowing any concern to drift from your mind. Now repeat gently to yourself, "My life is full of peace and happiness. Today is a perfect day."

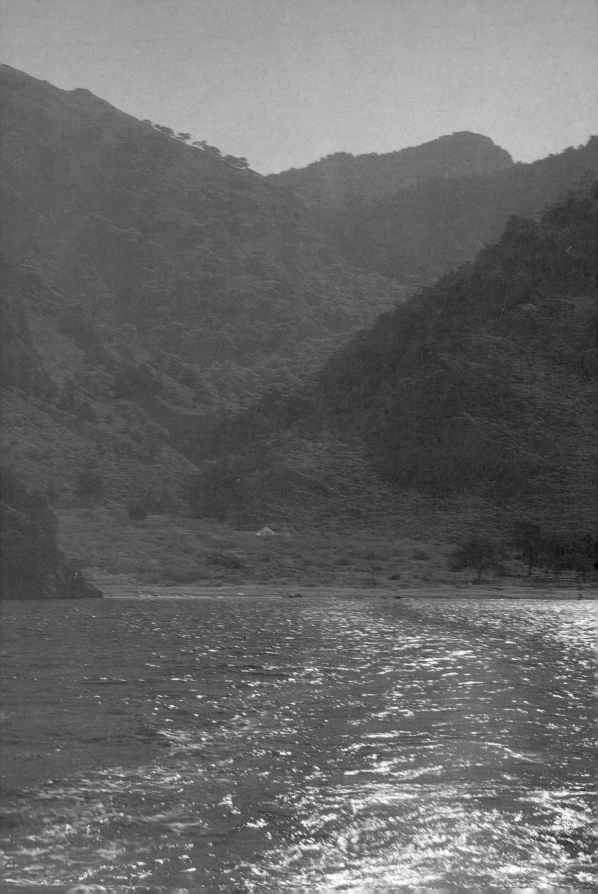

Environment

Toxic substances impinge on everything you do, from your eating and sleeping habits, to leisure or employment. Some toxins are inescapable, but there is a lot you can do to lessen your exposure and mitigate the effects. This section will help you to identify more precisely just what you can avoid and how you can protect yourself as you go about your daily business.

Any part of your environment can offer potential dangers or toxins, from obvious pollutants like untreated sewage on the beach or chemical contamination of river water, to the very air you breathe: it may carry toxins, or be too humid, too dry, too hot or cold, or contain too many positive ions in it for our good.

Tap water in industrialized countries almost always contains toxic substances. And even if you were to have your own, uncontaminated well, the pipes carrying the water might poison it.

Sunlight itself is an irritant in anything but small doses, and artificial light usually carries hazards as well.

And many toxic substances, some exceedingly nasty, may lurk in your home or place of work (p.28-9).

By becoming aware of potential toxic danger, whether at home, on your way to work or the shops, travelling – even going on holiday, and while you are there – you can make a start on raising the quality of your own environment. This awareness makes a great deal of sense, if you intend applying detoxification principles to your life, ridding your body of what is already affecting it, and protecting it against future exposure to toxicity.

These pages (114-129) will describe the air in your home and work-place, and the positive steps you can take to get it as health-enhancing as possible. You will, for example, find strategies for getting your water supply fit to drink, and information on the safety and labelling of bottled waters. There is also a recipe of special nutrients, mixed in the kitchen, which can, if taken regularly, assist the safe removal of heavy metals from your body. You may already have acquired these from water, or other sources, such as mercury lurking in the fillings in your teeth and causing toxic reactions. The importance of full-spectrum light as a nutrient is revealed, and the consequences of this for health bring light within the scope of your detoxification programme, along with the hazards and safety measures associated with radiation.

You can do much to improve your own health by improving the "health" of the buildings you live and work in, and the good character of your shopping list of "essentials" for cleaning, maintenance or decorating. This spring-cleaned, non-toxic shopping list extends to hygiene and cosmetic products as well.

In the kitchen, you have some choice of equipment and cooking methods both to avoid obvious contamination and to safeguard such nutrients as your food retains before you begin the preparation process. This process is, of course, only the final stage in the series that brings food to your table. It is suggested here that you lean toward the organic in whatever you buy.

Air

Clean, healthy air makes all the difference to the way you feel, and it is not just the absence of pollutants that determines its quality. Pressure, temperature and humidity, the amount of movement, the content of positive and negative ions – all need to be present at optimum levels for optimum wellbeing.

Pollutants   Most modern city dwellers spend 90 percent of their time indoors, where fumes from copying machines, cleaning solvents, and modern building materials, and risks from bug-infested air conditioning systems can seriously – even fatally – damage health. Efficient, well-serviced, non-polluting machines for air control, plus getting fresh air into the home or work place, are the keys to healthy air.

Outdoors, short of wearing face-masks, there is little you can do to avoid air pollution except keep away from heavy traffic, dry-cleaning or hairdressing premises in town.

Humidity   Double glazing and mechanical heating lower humidity levels dangerously. This can lead to respiratory distress as the delicate mucous membranes of the nose, eyes and throat dry out, leading to infections, feelings of tiredness, restlessness, insomnia and vague, flu-like symptoms. Improve matters by buying a humidifier or indoor plants: they give off water into the atmosphere by transpiration.

Air movement   If you cannot open a window, or the air-conditioner recycles stale air, you will feel lethargic and light-headed. If no other choice is available, go outside for a walk frequently during the day.

Temperature   Most modern homes and workplaces are too hot. 68°F (20°C) is optimum temperature for physical work; a 15 percent reduction in efficiency results at 75°F (24°C); 61°F (16°C) is best for mental work.

Pressure   Rapid changes in pressure can trigger off unpleasant symptoms. Conditions such as rheumatism, depression, TB, asthma and anxiety are aggravated by the drop in pressure that heralds a storm.

Ions   The air is alive with positively and negatively charged electrical particles which enter the body through skin or lungs. In general we are more alert when negative ions are high and feel unwell when positive ions predominate.

Negative ions make you feel energetic and vital, enhance sporting prowess, improve productivity and reduce all symptoms of ill-health present. They are increased:
* in seaside or mountain air;
* after a storm;
* by ioniser machines.

Positive ions make you feel fatigued and heavy, inattentive and unproductive. They are increased:
* before storms;
* when warm prevailing winds blow;
* during periods of sun-spot activity;
* by high levels of natural radioactivity in the soil;
* by synthetic materials, smoke, chemical fumes;
* by all mechanical and electrical activity in machinery, including computers and air conditioning.

A negative/positive ratio of 12 : 10 is thought to be ideal.

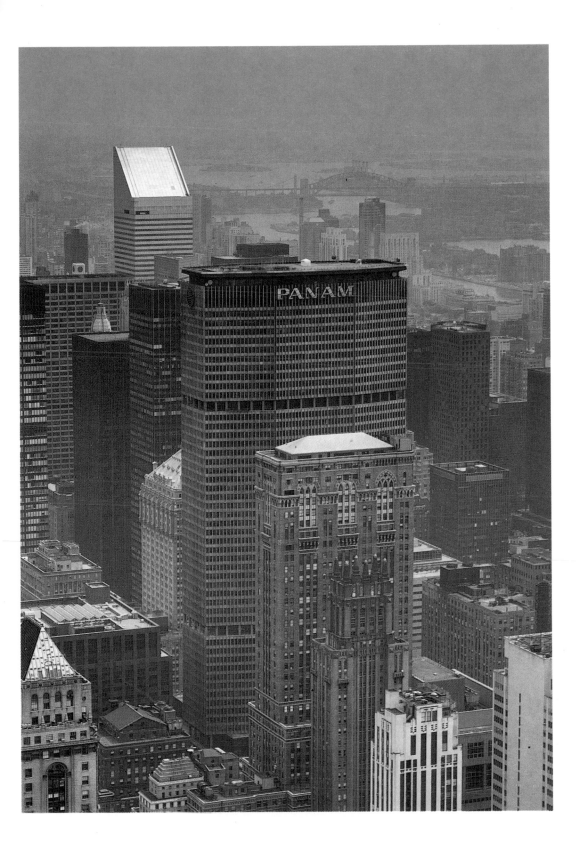

Water

Our bodies enjoy a peculiarly intimate relationship with water: 80 percent of their volume consists of this vital element which requires constant topping up. Water transports nutrients, helps regulate body temperature, acts as a solvent in the digestive process, and assists in waste removal. You quite literally have to drink to live.

Pure water has no toxicity at all, and yet water is potentially one of your most likely sources of toxins. Much tap water is recycled, so last night's bathwater may cook tomorrow's vegetables. Water supplies can contain a cocktail of ingredients, some by accident, such as surplus agricultural nitrates and pesticides, washed into the soil and so into the system, and others by design, such as chlorine (to kill bacteria), aluminium (as aluminium sulphate it is added to settle out solid impurities) and fluoride (to reduce tooth decay). Nitrates are particularly dangerous to babies; aluminium is implicated in premature senile dementia (Alzheimer's disease), and fluoride in a range of health problems from allergic reaction to cancer, and even cot death. These and the hundreds of synthetic organic chemicals also found as traces in drinking water are strongly suspected of being carcinogenic or mutagenic.

Lead, leached into the water from pipes, accumulates in the body, interferes with vital enzyme functions and affects, particularly, the intellectual development of children. There is no safe level of lead.

What can you do about water toxicity? Get the public health officer to test your water. Check your pipework. Run the tap for several minutes first thing in the morning. Filter tap water for drinking and cooking. Shower or bathe quickly if your water is contaminated.

Simple water filter jugs and tap devices remove chlorine, lime, some organic chemicals and bacteria, but for higher-quality water you will need a more sophisticated system. Different methods remove different substances:

Reverse osmosis filtration removes salts and sediments but does not cope with inorganic chemicals such as lead.

Carbon filtration is effective for organic and inorganic substances; it does not remove calcium or magnesium.

Distillation kills bacteria and extracts dissolved solids and trace metals. With an extra carbon filter to remove organics, this is the most efficient method.

Water softeners remove excessive levels of calcium and magnesium, but the added sodium is bad for both blood pressure and cardiovascular health.

Did you know
– that nitrates which enter our water supply from fertilizers used in farming cause "blue baby" syndrome in infants, and may cause cancer of the bowel in adults?
– that four million people in the UK drink water with nitrate levels above the European safety limits (50mg per litre)?
– that an excessive amount of aluminium sulphate, added to purify water, will turn your hair green? It is a neurotoxin and has been linked to the development of premature senile dementia (Alzheimer's disease).

Oral chelation

Chelation comes from the Greek word which means to "claw", describing the action of some nutrients which can literally "grab hold" of unwanted toxic substances and help them on their way out of your body. An example of this is oatmeal which does this with cholesterol and some toxic metals. Make up a week's supply of chelation mixture (recipe right), store it in the refrigerator and eat it with breakfast.

A gram of amino acids (either cysteine or methionine) taken daily away from mealtimes will help if you have heavy metal toxicity.

● Teeth fillings

Mercury is probably the most toxic metal to which we are exposed – and most of us have large amounts of it in the amalgam fillings in our teeth. We now know this gradually leaches into the body, either dissolved in saliva, escaping as gas, or passing along nerve roots directly to the brain. It affects the nervous system, sometimes resulting in numbness, extreme fatigue, mental incapacity and even paralysis. Amalgam combinations now being used are even more toxic than before. Sweden, the first country to tackle the problem, has banned amalgam fillings in pregnant women.

Don't have your teeth filled with amalgam; when you can, replace existing amalgams with porcelain, gold or plastic. If you have high mercury levels (you can test this: the small ads in health magazines will direct you to hair analysis laboratories), use the chelation formula and take additional high doses of vitamin C.

Oral chelation mixture
* 28g lecithin granules and 84g coarsely chopped sunflower seeds (for lineolic acid, zinc and potassium);
* 35g brewer's yeast (B vitamins, selenium and chromium);
* 14g bone meal (calcium and magnesium);
* 35g wheatgerm (vitamin E);
* 3500mg vitamin C (as powdered sodium ascorbate);
* 700iu vitamin E (empty a capsule);
* 175mg zinc (as zinc gluconate or picolinate).

(iu = international unit
1oz = 28.35grams)

Bottled water

Any bottled spring water is likely to be better for you than any tap water, but there is variation: some will suit you better than others.

Most labels carry information about calcium (Ca), magnesium (Mg), potassium (K), sodium (Na), sulphates (SO_4), chlorides (Cl), nitrates (NO_3), fluoride (F), bicarbonates (HCO_3), and acidity/alkalinity (pH). Quantities are usually expressed in milligrams (mg) per litre (l), but also milligrams per 100 millilitres (mg/100ml: multiply figure by ten for comparability) or parts per million (ppm).

Look for reasonably high levels of calcium and magnesium; they make the water "hard" (good for your heart). Avoid high levels of sodium (bad for your blood pressure). Keep levels of sulphates, chlorides, nitrates and fluorides low.

The pH reading signifies the acidity of the water. Neutral is pH 7.0. Acidic water (low pH number) will leach chemicals from water pipes and plastic bottles. A neutral or higher reading is therefore desirable.

Light as a nutrient

The retina of the eye contains photosensitive receptor cells which work independently of the optical system. They convert light energy into chemical energy and transmit messages via the nervous system to the pineal and pituitary glands which control the hormonal system of the body. Natural light is vital to physical wellbeing.

The entire electromagnetic spectrum is contained in sunlight, and this light is as much a nutrient to the body as any food. Deprived of this full-spectrum light adverse changes in health and function take place, including Seasonal Affective Disorders (SAD) which cause severe depression in winter.

Behaviour is altered in deficient light. One researcher studied a group of Florida first-grade schoolchildren under standard cool white fluorescent light. They displayed evidence of nervous fatigue, irritability, attention lapses and hyperactive behaviour. When moved to full-spectrum lighting, behaviour improved, nervousness lessened and classroom performance improved. Even the incidence of cavities in their teeth was lowered.

Other evidence of light's powerful influence includes the facts that:
* Infants with jaundice improve when full-spectrum lighting stimulates the body to excrete toxic wastes through the skin and kidneys more efficiently.
* Muscle strength is enhanced under full-spectrum light. Dr John Ott's research points to the beneficial effect of full-spectrum lighting in maternity hospitals on reducing the need for caesarean sections. He also estimates that we lose about half the strength available from muscles when we are behind glass. Even with sunglasses, pink and orange cause greater weakness than blue lenses because of the wavelengths they screen.

Incandescent light (from ordinary light bulbs) contains virtually no ultra- violet and is deficient at the blue end of the visible light spectrum. Fluorescent tube light is even more distorted, particularly at the red end of the spectrum. Full-spectrum lamps more closely resemble the spectral balance of daylight and its ultra-violet but, while low levels of exposure to ultraviolet is considered beneficial, depletion of the ozone layer allows greater penetration of high-energy radiation (UV-C) and gives rise to concern. Those susceptible to skin cancer, or people who are especially vulnerable to radiation in some other way (children in particular) need to be protected.

To make the benefits of full-spectrum light available,
1 Install windows, sliding doors and skylights made of
ultraviolet- transmitting plastic (UVP). Many dealers are
unaware of the difference, but all can order it. Now become
aware of the dangers of *over*-exposure.
2 Get ultraviolet-transmitting spectacle or contact lenses in
clear or neutral gray glass or plastic from an optician; they
allow even filtration without distortion of the light spectrum.
People who have had surgery for cataracts will need medical advice about this.
3 Install full-spectrum artificial light in your home and, if
possible, place of work. Make sure fluorescent tubes,
whether full-spectrum or not, are fully shielded as some
radiation is given off. Use daylight incandescent bulbs
where fluorescent tubes are inappropriate.
4 Get out of doors, or at least sit by an open window, for at
least an hour a day. It is not necessary to be in full sunlight to
obtain the benefits of light. You will have access to the full
range of light waves sitting in the shade of a porch or under
a tree, provided you are not using glasses or lenses. Use
glasses or lenses outdoors as little as possible.

Avoid radiation hazards associated with sunbathing where
possible and in any case between 10am and 3pm when they
are greatest. Beware also of artificial sun-tanning: any
machines which require you to wear goggles are likely to be
a source of short-wave ultraviolet rays. This harmful end of
the spectrum is very close to X-ray radiation and, in natural
sunlight, should be filtered out by the ozone layer.

Full-spectrum lamps more
closely resemble the spectral
balance of daylight than do
either fluorescent tubes or incandescent lamps.

The lamps (ordinary light-
bulbs) are ultra-violet deficient
and heavily weighted towards
the infrared end of the visible
light spectrum, producing a
high proportion of heat.

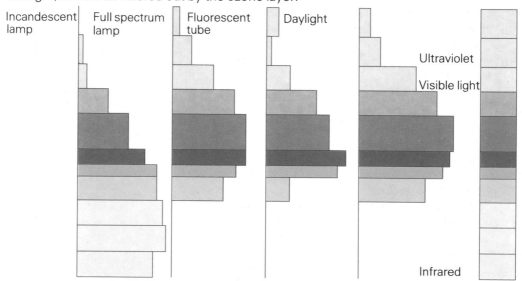

| Incandescent lamp | Full spectrum lamp | Fluorescent tube | Daylight |

Ultraviolet

Visible light

Infrared

Radiation

We are exposed to radiation throughout life. Most (90 percent) is naturally occurring: it reaches us from space, or is released by the breakdown of radioactive substances in the earth, such as radon gas from uranium in the bedrock. Some is the byproduct of modern industry and technology: a choice for desirables such as electric power is often a choice for undesirables such as the thorium, radium and polonium pumped out of coal-burning power stations.

Our bodies are designed to cope with a certain level of ambient radiation. Although in strict terms there is no such thing as a harmless dose, we are radiation-tolerant up to a point. Beyond this point the body cannot repair the damage caused to its cells, and it is the young, going through their growth period, or people suffering other forms of stress, who are particularly vulnerable.

High level (ionising) radiation damages the genetic material in cells and can make them malignant. It also alters the ability of the body to regenerate its tissues through normal protein synthesis, and dramatically speeds up the ageing process. These effects depend on many interacting elements, such as the strength of the radiation, the length of exposure and the amount the body absorbs. This last factor is expressed as REMs (radiation equivalent in man) when specifically related to humans.

Average annual exposure in the US and Western Europe is between 100 and 200 millirems (1000 millirems = 1 rem). At exposure levels of 25 rems a year serious blood changes take place; above 100 rems, fatigue, weakness, loss of hair and some digestive problems, mostly reversible. 200 rems can produce infertility. At 400 rems, half of those exposed die; at 600 rems everyone dies. (Bacteria and insects are more resistant: it takes 50,000 rems to kill bacteria when irradiating food.)

Whether we like it or not, we may even be exposed to radiation in the sanctuary of our own homes. About half the natural radiation exposure, overall, is from radon gas which occurs in rocks in certain areas. It leaks slowly into houses or is carried there by water passing through natural rock formations, especially granite, en route to our taps and showers. Radon may also be present, at lower levels, in building blocks and concrete (50 percent more than in wooden) houses; cement also contains high levels of uranium and thorium. It is extremely important to try to clear these avoidable hazards out of the house (see p.122-3).

Computer screens
The terminal screen carries a positive ion charge which pulls positive ions towards it, leading to an unhealthy local environment. Anti-glare protective screens are available which can reduce this effect and eliminate static electricity. Sit at least 20 inches away and take frequent fresh-air breaks. Pregnant women should avoid lengthy periods near a monitor.

An average intake above which ill-effects are noted is thought to be 5000 mrems (5 rems) a year for adults and 100 mrems for still-growing teenagers; young children are even more susceptible.

1 rem of radiation adds 50 percent to the chances of a child's developing cancer before puberty.

Avoid X-rays during pregnancy.

Healthy room

There is some evidence that the risk from pollutants in modern homes and offices approaches that from radiation or toxic chemicals in industry. There is quite a lot you can do to minimise this risk by making informed choices in furnishings and equipment and taking certain evasive action. If, for example, you suspect you may live in a radon-producing area or home, you can immediately seek professional assessment, and get the radon source sealed off from the home, and vented away.

Bring fresh air into the living or work space; introduce ionisers and humidifiers; choose carpets, curtains and furnishings of natural fibre; be lavish with plants. They do sterling work in enhancing environmental health.

Furnishings: use wood not plastic; wool, silk and cotton, not synthetics; clay or ceramic tiles and slate not concrete, plastic or composites.

Machinery: place ionisers wherever there is electrical equipment e.g. cookers, washing machines, TV. Air conditioning may call for humidifiers as well; regularly clean and check filters.

Windows: if you cannot open some each day, insist on fresh air intake ducts from the outside world. Make sure these are kept free from mould or bacteria.

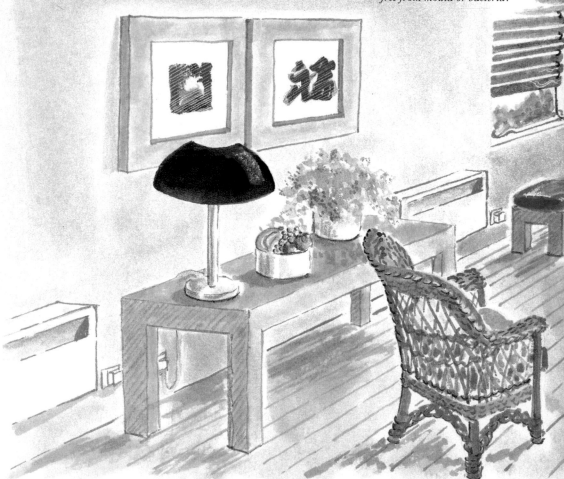

Plants: choose green plants to absorb carbon dioxide; allaomena and syndonium to take up benzene fumes, and philodendron and spider plants to extract large amounts of formaldehyde from the atmosphere. Be extravagant.

Wall or roof insulation material may give off formaldehyde or other chemical vapours. Get professional advice to counteract, vent or neutralise this.

Lighting: introduce full-spectrum lighting wherever you spend a lot of time.

Heating: check solid fuel, gas, or oil boilers for fumes and ventilate correctly. Electric heating is cleaner.

Walls: avoid synthetic coverings and panelling. Use natural paper, non-toxic paint or wood.

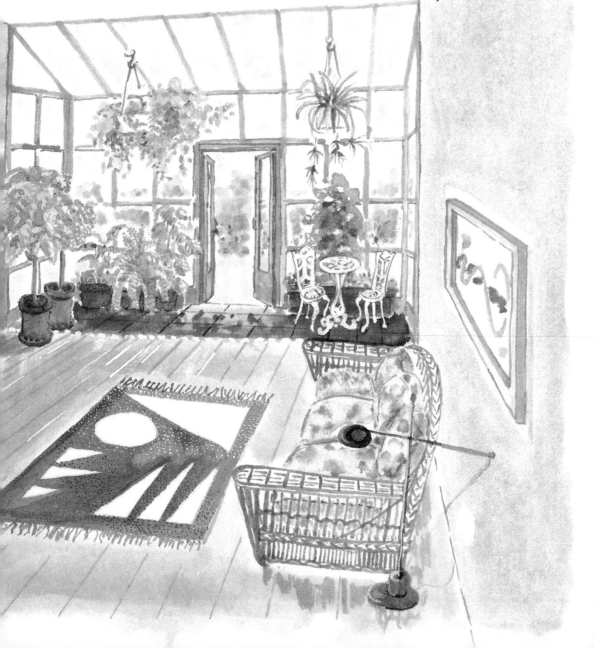

Danger lurks in all sorts of surprising places. We might expect some sort of risk from nuclear power stations (in fact they are reasonably safe, provided they do not leak; the main problem is in the disposal of waste materials, and the vulnerable operations of commissioning and decommissioning); but consider some less obvious areas:

* Many optical glasses are radioactive: the rare earths used to produce them contain thorium or uranium and may produce cataracts. Fit plastic lenses.
* The white mantles of campers' lamps are highly radioactive (thorium again) with emission highest soon after lighting. Light and leave outdoors for 20 minutes before bringing lamp into a confined space; wash hands well.
* Many fertilizers used in gardening or agriculture contain radioactive phosphates. Use organic composts.
* Many ceramic and glassware materials in household utensils contain uranium oxide which produces high energy gamma radiation. Most suspect are those orange, red, beige or yellow pots with a highly reflective surface.
* Thirty cigarettes a day expose a smoker to the same degree of radiation as someone who has three *hundred* chest X-rays a year (15 rems). The broad tobacco leaf attracts radioactive polonium, and lead 210 from, it is thought, the phosphate-based fertilizers used in its cultivation. Lead 210 is known to remain in the lung for years, or migrate to other tissues, emitting radiation constantly. This danger extends to passive smokers too.
* The higher we fly (or climb), the thinner the air, the more radiation from the cosmos. This is thought to be a factor contributing to "jet lag".

● **Protective measures**
1 Avoid obvious sources (see above).
2 Take antioxidant nutrients (see box) to protect against damage.
3 Use foods with high fibre content which specifically help extract radioactive materials from the digestive system: apples, pears, sunflower and pumpkin seeds for pectin, seaweed for algin, oatmeal for natural fibre. Calcium (up to 1500 mg daily in divided doses in tablet form, or from vegetables and apples) also competes with strontium or cesium in the bowel, preventing at least some of it from entering the bloodstream.

Vast amounts of low level radiation are emitted by computer terminal display screens, telecommunication machines, and old fashioned colour TVs. It does not produce the cellular damage of high level radiation, but is thought to be a constant irritant to our chemical communication systems (enzymes) and also to our nervous system.

Radiation damage is affected by overall health and nutritional status. Ensure adequate levels of antioxidant nutrients such as the vitamins A, C, E, the mineral selenium, and amino acids such as cysteine and methionine.

The highest scorers are likely to be:
* Anyone working in nuclear power generation.
* Coal miners or anyone working in power generation from coal.
* Medical or dental X-ray and radiotherapy personnel.
* Anyone working in research, production or frequent use of cement or concrete, gypsum, anhydride, ceramics, optical glass, phosphorus fertilizers, tobacco, campers' lamps, smoke detectors, luminous watch dials or any other source of radiation.
* Airline crew or frequent flyers.
* Smokers and those who live and work with them.
* People whose homes are built on radon-rich rock or over underground water sources.

Jet lag strategy
Take tablets of the anti-oxidant enzymes gluta-thione peroxidase, super oxide dismutase (SOD), catalase and/or methionine reductase before and during flight with plenty of fluid (not alcohol) or vitamins C and E at maximum recommended levels.

Nuclear weapon test fallout
4.4 mrem

Cosmic rays
35 mrem

Thirty cigarettes a day
1500 mrem

Radioactive decay
(e.g. carbon 14, potassium 40)
27 mrem

Medical diagnosis
70 mrem

Energy production sources
(e.g. electricity) 3 mrem

Radiation from soil
35 mrem

Radiation exposure of average US citizen

What high scorers should do:
Eat foods which contain (or take regular supplements of):
Beta-carotene (orange, yellow, red fruits and vegetables

Vitamin E (wheatgerm)
Vitamin C (all green vegetables, salads, fruits)
Amino acid cysteine
Selenium (garlic)
Evening primrose oils
Kelp tablets (iodine and algin)

Daily supplement dose

25 milligrams

200 i.u.
½ to 3 grams

1 to 3 grams
200 micrograms
½ to 1 gram
3 to 6 tablets

These are all available from health stores or pharmacists. Except for cysteine, take with food.

Household products

The products we are accustomed to using for cleaning, polishing, maintenance or decorating have all, generally, been potentially highly toxic. Most contain a wide range of volatile toxic chemicals such as ammonia, turpentine, naphthalene, acetone, chlorine and benzene. All cause irritation on contact with skin or eyes and, if inhaled, produce damage to tissues.

As the green movement gathers momentum, however, safer alternatives are reaching the market. For instance, consumer awareness of the presence of the dreadfully toxic dioxin in all bleached paper, has resulted in unbleached paper products now outselling bleached in Scandinavia. Similar consumer revolutions are taking place throughout Europe and starting in the US.

As a first step, become aware of specific dangers. Aerosol sprays, whatever their purpose, are among the nastiest sources of toxic chemicals. While some are being phased out because of the damage their propellants do to the ozone layer, the fine mist of chemicals they all dispense damages you as you inhale and absorb it.

Dyes, paints and solvent cleaners contain a wide array of highly dangerous substances. Paint strippers and solvents often contain known cancer-causing agents. Metal paints are particularly hazardous: undesirable metals are easily absorbed through the skin. Water-based paints are safer than plastic. Prefer traditional non-chemical glues or water-based acrylics with a low solvent content. Chemicals which kill insects, rats and mice are often lethal to humans as well; garden fertilizers and sprays present similar if lesser hazards. Use organic alternatives wherever possible.

Avoid composite "woods" such as chipboard, hardboard and ply which give off formaldehyde and other toxic vapours, and the highly toxic fungicides, pesticides and contact chemicals used in treating timber. Choose instead solid wood (not tropical, if you wish to conserve rain forests), bamboo, wicker or rattan, or older, recycled timber. Try for preservatives, stains and sealants that are non-toxic wherever available.

Avoid plastics. Their complex toxic content often contaminates whatever they touch, and the environment around them. Avoid also foam-filled cushions and upholstery, using feathers, down, and horse-hair, covered with cotton, hessian, wool or other natural fibres.

Strategies for safety
Avoid what obviously upsets you

Use protective gloves and masks

Seek hard for safer alternatives

Give your protective mechanisms (enzymes) a head start with high standards of nutritional excellence

Toxic exposure
The interior of a new car contains the vapours of over 100 different chemicals, many of them highly toxic, including formaldehyde, phenolic compounds and organo-chlorines.

Anyone decorating the home with modern petro-chemical based paints and solvents is exposed to even greater toxicity.

Soap, oral hygiene and cosmetics

Almost any paste, powder or lotion applied to the skin can be absorbed through it and affect the internal tissues and organs of the body, as well as the skin itself. It is crucial, therefore, to choose the products you are going to rub into yourself with exquisite care.

To loosen dead skin cells, degrease the skin and remove dirt, soap needs to be slightly alkaline. Unfortunately the more alkaline it is – and most commercial soaps are extremely alkaline – the more damage it does to the sensitive balance of the skin's ecology (healthy skin is slightly acidic, thanks to the natural secretions which protect and lubricate it) by allowing easy access to bacteria. Soaps which are only slightly alkaline are those containing glycerine or olive oil, or those made with oatmeal, aloe or other vegetable bases. Restore natural acidity safely after washing by rinsing with cider vinegar.

Cosmetics are the source of an extremely wide variety of potentially dangerous allergens and highly toxic chemicals. You should, at least, not use cosmetic products which have any sort of warning on the label; it is there for good reason. Choose one of the new, safer, often herb-based, products that are now available. Bear in mind, though, that the inclusion of a herb does not itself exclude undesirable chemicals nor guarantee that the herbal extract itself is not an irritant. Or you could make your own: a number of fine, herbal beauty books are on the market to show you how to make safe, pure products from flowers, plants and other natural ingredients.

Active encouragement of the horribly cruel use of animals in the allergen testing of most commercial cosmetics can now be ended by buying products which clearly state that they have not used such methods.

Some of the chemicals which find their way into our mouths via toothpastes and mouthwashes are quite outrageous: ammonia, ethanol, and formaldehyde, to name but a few. For sweet breath it is necessary only to remove decaying food particles by brushing or flossing. Herb-based pastes can be used in preference to the abrasive and chemically dubious commercial offerings. Bacteria will be discouraged by plaque removal: you could use fine sea-salt and finish by rubbing the teeth with a fresh herb such as sage. A soft brush with round natural bristles used at all angles – not just up and down – also helps massage the gums, reducing risk of periodontal gum disease, one of the commonest diseases around.

Hexachlorophene, an antibacterial agent once widely used in soaps, is now restricted to prescription compounds only: in the mid-1970s 39 babies died in the US as a result of its proven ability to enter the bloodstream, attack nerve cells and cause irreversible brain damage.

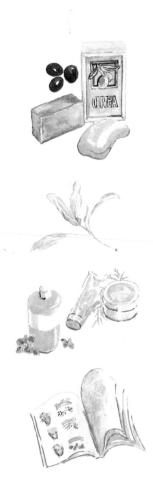

Storing and cooking food

Plastic containers for food storage can add to your toxic burden. The volatile chemical constituents, especially in non-rigid plastics ("thermo-plastics") are likely to contaminate whatever is stored, or in the case of cling-film, cooked in it. Look out for "plasticiser-free" cling-film which overcomes this difficulty. The process of cooking some foods in a plastic bag is potentially highly toxic, and soft drinks such as colas, lemonades, fruit drinks or mineral waters supplied in plastic bottles are almost always chemically contaminated. Choose clay, china, porcelain or, of course, glass containers.

Glass is the safest material for cooking – though, as a poor conductor of heat, not the most efficient. Disadvantages are attached to almost all others:

* Aluminium is to be avoided (see p.116). Both utensils and foil wrappings can add this highly dangerous substance to food cooked or stored in them, especially acidic foods such as fruit, tomato sauce, wine or vinegar.
* Copper utensils have to be lined with unscratched stainless steel to prevent the copper entering the food chain with serious toxic consequences. Discard any pots if the steel lining is scratched.
* Cast iron vessels certainly allow iron to enter the food cooked in them. This may be beneficial, but excessive levels can crowd out intake of other vital nutrients such as zinc, leading to deficiency.
* Non-stick (teflon-coated) pans are also sources of minute quantities of toxic by-products. Use them sparingly.
* Stainless steel is a fine cooking medium. It must be unscratched; see *copper* above.
* High quality enamel is safe. Cheaper utensils may contain toxic oxides which leach into food.
* Clay pottery containers are reckoned to be safe unless glazed, as happens, with lead or cadmium.

The best cooking methods are judged by the level of nutrients left at the end of the day. Steaming, stir-frying and pressure cooking all rate highly by this criterion, and the enzymes inevitably lost by microwave cooking can be replaced by increasing the amount of raw food eaten.

Check microwave ovens regularly: leakage is a radiation hazard. Make sure the whole kitchen is well-ventilated. Cooking fumes may contain potentially carcinogenic substances such as benzopyrenes; charcoal-broiled or deep-fried foods are particularly risky.

If vegetables are placed in cold water and brought to the boil, more than half the vitamin C will be lost. Add vegetables to water that has already boiled off its vitamin-destructive oxygen content.

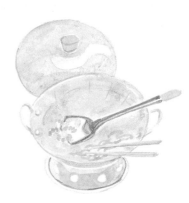

The shape of pots and pans is almost as important as the materials from which they are made. The deeper the pot the better it holds liquids, ideal for soups and stews. A shallow skillet or wok, on the other hand, is ideal for stir-frying, allowing the food to lose liquid through evaporation and contact with air, producing a "drier" food. In micro-wave cooking a different principle applies, the heat being generated at the centre of the food rather than being applied to its outside surface.

Food and depleted food

A major dilemma of modern times is consumer demand for safe, nutritious food, freshly available at all times. This is just not possible without some loss of food value, due at the very least to the time lag between farm and table. We have always had to process food: even wholemeal products, for example, are altered from their original whole grain form; but how far are we prepared to go down the path of refining food to the point of sterility and nutritional decadence?

Part of the modern imperative rests on commercial considerations of storage and adequate shelf-life. These often dictate the removal of essential nutrients or the addition of preservatives and stabilizers. However, excessive use of colouring, pesticides, fungicides and other additives which owe their inclusion to "consumer appeal" may not be quite so necessary. While we may have to compromise our purist principles a bit, or else grow our own food, we can certainly try to educate suppliers, and ease the toxic burden on our bodies, by simply not buying over-processed foods.

Read labels carefully. Be aware of E- additives; plenty of good printed listings are available. Search out meat, poultry or fish that is free of hormone or antibiotic contamination. (This will often mean finding free-ranging food-animals, including game.) Shop around: wholefood stores generally stock excellent products; and supermarket chains are increasingly aware of the commercial wisdom of stocking organic and free range goods.

Irradiation is a new development for increased shelf-life. This process, which kills dangerous bacteria such as salmonella (though not the deadly botulinus toxin), destroys the very elements in the food which, from a nutritional point of view, make it most worth eating, its enzymes, and most of the vitamin E. Other casualties are the micro-organisms which warn by their putrid smell when food is going off, and the yeasts and moulds which, by competing with bacteria, provide a natural control on their growth. Not affected by irradiation, absurdly enough, are the chemical poisons (toxins) created by bacteria contamination which are the real health hazard.

Ensuring a healthy balance between the loss of essential nutrients in processing and cooking, and the enjoyment of delicious food, is a dilemma. Most people living in industrialized societies have deficiences of at least one essential nutrient (over 40 are needed for good health). A prudent strategy should involve good food selection, sound cooking methods and safe vitamin/mineral supplementation.

The toxic effects of white sugar are so widespread – sugar lacks nutrients, depresses the immune system, contributes to tooth decay, obesity, diabetes, heart disease, migraine headaches, psychological disorders, yeast overgrowth – that Prof. Yudkin of London University says, "If only a small fraction of what is known about the effects of sugar were revealed in relation to any other food additive, that material would promptly be banned".

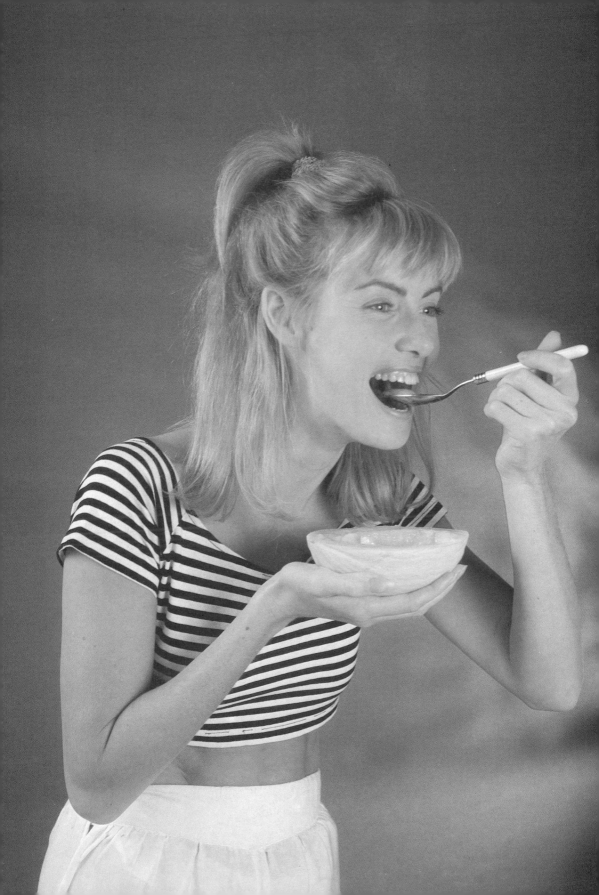

Diet and fasting

What you eat can kill or cure you. This is not just the view of fruit and nut case "cranks" who have, of course, been saying this for years, but even of the World Health Organisation. All major medical and governmental agencies now agree, for instance, that sorting out problems which stem from dietary imbalances (deficiencies, unbalanced ratios – for example, in the type of fats described on p.132 – as well as toxicities) would reduce the incidence of cancer enormously; a staggering 80 percent of cancers are now known to have at least part of their cause in the area of nutrition. Together, environmental toxicities and hazards (radiation, for example) and nutrition account for the causes of most cancers, almost all of which are, therefore, potentially preventable. The same is true of cardiovascular disease, and there is a strong suspicion that diet is similarly involved in many other chronic degenerative diseases, including arthritis.

The major killer diseases of Western society are related, sometimes intimately, to our daily eating habits: how much fat (and of what kind) we eat, how much or how little fresh vegetable, whether we choose red meat or opt for a vegetarian or fish diet. Good diet is a matter of getting a right balance of proteins, fats, carbohydrates, minerals, vitamins and fibre. Achieving a "balanced diet" is a major part of long-term detoxification.

By taking personal responsibility for your own health, through diet as well as lifestyle and other habits, you can do a great deal to promote present wellbeing and to prevent long-term degeneration.

Most people in developed countries are free to make this choice for health. You can, firstly, reject foods which add to the toxic load and, secondly, decide in favour of dietary strategies to boost intake of anti-oxidant and energy-raising nutrients that improve immune function and actually encourage detoxification.

Research into the individual powers of some amino acids, for example, has shown that, by careful selection of foods or by specific supplementation, it is possible to alter the biochemical environment of the brain, increase powers of concentration and encourage a more relaxed and positive attitude to life.

Greater energy, heightened health, better overall physical function, increased resistance to illness (infection as well as chronic disease), clearer mental functioning – correct eating can deliver all these benefits. And it can be fun: you don't have to spend your life anxiously weighing every morsel before you swallow it. On the contrary: once you understand the balances necessary, the major damaging factors and the most important principles, you will find a wide range of personal choice which takes account of taste and social needs as well as cost.

Within the framework of sound nutrition described in this chapter, you can devise a programme of regular periods of inner cleansing, detoxification (fasting, mono-diets, raw food days) without the need to disrupt your life too much, or of becoming deficient in the process. If, however, you recognise yourself in this photograph; or, if you are eating uncontrollably; or if you are not eating as much as people are telling you you should, then first seek advice from health or nutrition professionals.

A *basic diet*

Protein Depending on your age and energy output you will need to eat between 3 and 5 ounces (85 – 140 grams) of first-class protein daily. First class protein is derived from animal sources and contains all the amino acids your body needs to make new tissue. If you do not eat animal derivatives, these amino acids must be obtained from vegetable sources. (See p.85.)

Fats In order to survive we need a source of essential fatty acids. The right proportion of fats and oils is between 25 and 30 percent of our daily calorie intake. People who eat up to 40 percent of their food from these sources, in the West they are the majority, are at risk from cancer and heart disease.

Fats are either saturated (mainly animal products), poly-unsaturated (margarine, sunflower oil) or monounsaturated (olive oil). The more the carbon atoms in fatty acids are linked to hydrogen, the more "saturated" the fat or oil is said to be. Our interest in saturation relates largely to its effect on cholesterol, a waxy substance vital to cell life but dangerous to heart health in excess. In general, saturated fats raise cholesterol levels in the blood; polyunsaturates reduce all forms of it, including the beneficial high density form, while monounsaturated oils reduce only the harmful low and very low density lipoprotein fractions of cholesterol.

Carbohydrates We need the complex carbodyhdrates in fruits, vegetables, nuts, seeds, beans and grains for their protective vitamin, mineral, enzyme and fibre content. Once these foods have been processed and refined, however, they lose at least some, and often almost all, of their useful detoxifying nutrients.

The combining of certain food "families" can be helpful in aiding digestion. The opposite is also true: some combinations are thought to be undesirable in that they can cause digestive problems and incomplete digestion.

(Note: there is general but not total agreement amongst experts on which food combinations are "good" and which "bad". These are based on the author's personal experience and research.)

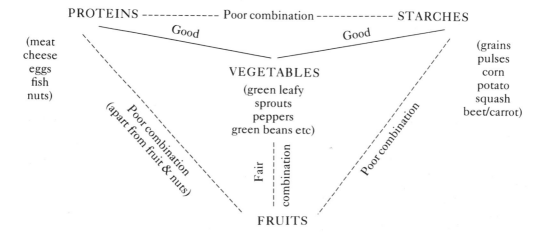

7 Day normal, basic diet menu

Day One
Breakfast: Oatmeal porridge, natural (live) yoghurt, one item of fresh fruit; drink herbal tea.
Lunch: Vegetable or bean soup and wholegrain bread. Side salad.
Supper: Grilled fish and steamed or stir-fried vegetables. Side salad.

Day Two
Breakfast: Fresh fruit, e.g. papaya, apple, grapes, or peach, and nuts.
Lunch: Cottage cheese salad and jacket potato.
Supper: Poultry or vegetarian savoury and vegetables.

Day Three
Breakfast: Homemade muesli (recipes on p.78) and fruit.
Lunch: Avocado salad with wholemeal bread and butter.
Supper: Omelette (mushroom, onion, tomato) and salad or vegetables.

Day Four
Breakfast: Natural (live) yoghurt, fresh fruit and nuts.
Lunch: Fresh tuna (or other fish) and salad or stir-fried vegetables.
Supper: Pasta and napolitano (tomato-based) sauce.

Day Five
Breakfast: Oatmeal porridge or homemade muesli, yoghurt, fruit.
Lunch: Vegetable or bean soup and wholegrain bread. Side salad.
Supper: Game, fish, poultry or vegetarian savoury and vegetables.

Day Six
Breakfast: Fresh fruit and nuts; yoghurt.
Lunch: Mixed salad, jacket potato and cottage cheese or avocado.
Supper: Grilled fish and steamed or stir-fried vegetables.

Day Seven
Breakfast: Boiled, poached or scrambled eggs, and rice cakes.
Lunch: Tomato and onion salad, and vegetarian savoury.
Supper: Soup and toast; fresh fruit; cheese.

Desserts: stewed or fresh fruit.
Drinks: between meals only. Choose bottled waters, some herbal teas (see p.138) or fruit juices. Restrict alcohol to a maximum of one glass of wine or half a pint of beer daily.

For good digestion:
* Do not drink with meals.
* Avoid very hot or very cold foods.
* Chew well: digestion, especially of carbohydrates, starts in the mouth.
* Don't eat if you are angry, upset or not hungry; have a rest or go for a walk instead.
* Don't eat different proteins (e.g. egg and meat) at one meal.
* Apply the combination principles opposite.

Iron is the most common "missing" nutrient world-wide. Nuts or wholegrains eaten with liver or meat, reduce your ability to absorb iron from these foods. A vitamin C-rich food at the same meal normalizes this process. Motto: eat green salad with every meal, especially those including grains and nuts.

Healthy cooking methods

To obtain maximum benefit from fruit and vegetables, eat them raw. However, cooking vegetables breaks down plant structures which are otherwise hard to digest, and releases the nutrients stored in them such as vitamins and minerals. This needs to be done carefully: overcooking destroys vitamins; throwing the boiling water away also throws out many of the minerals.

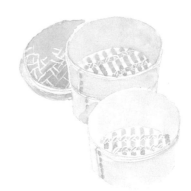

Steaming is a method which retains the maximum level of nutrients. Place the vegetables in a steamer or colander suspended over a pan of boiling water. They will be softened but still pleasantly crisp after just a few minutes.

Stir-Frying, in a traditional oriental wok, a high-sided, sloping container, is a healthy way to fry. Cut the food into small pieces; lightly oil the wok and put the pieces in when a high temperature is reached. The very hot oil seals the food surface, preventing fat absorption. Constantly agitate the food while cooking. It is ready when just slightly tenderized, retaining both nutrients and crispness.

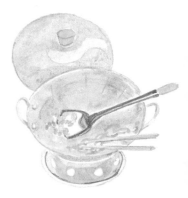

Baking in a traditional, unglazed, clay oven container helps to retain the maximum nutritional value and flavour (of fish or poultry in particular), and avoids the less desirable qualities of methods such as roasting or frying. Baking in clay containers produces an even distribution of heat, maintaining the food being cooked at a uniform temperature, preventing one part cooking at a faster rate than another. If vegetables are baked in this way, they slightly dehydrate but maintain their shape and flavour superbly. You can bake in containers made of other materials, but nothing compares with clay for results.

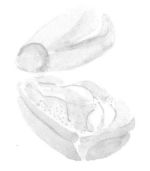

Temperature and Bacteria. Bacteria flourish and proliferate in the danger zone between 4.5°C and 60°C (40° and 140°F). Between 60°C and 75°C (140° and 167°F), growth is retarded. Most bacteria are destroyed at 100°C (212°F) (boiling point).

The common parasite, Toxoplasma gondii, found in meat from cattle, sheep and pigs, requires cooking for not less than 20 minutes at 80°C (176°F) or above to destroy it. Very little restaurant-cooked meat achieves anything like this, and fast food (such as hamburgers), never does.

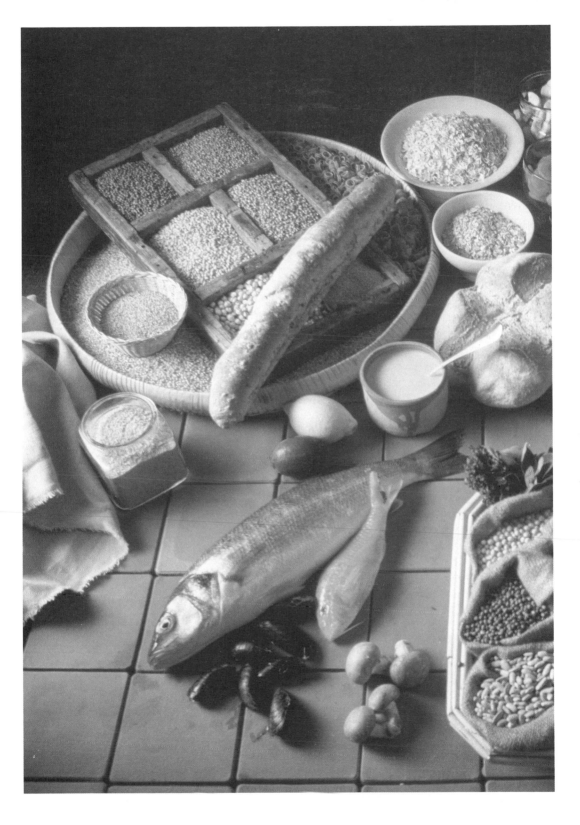

Special diets

● Food families

Foods fall into biological families. A person who is sensitive (allergic), to one member of a "family", is statistically more likely also to be sensitive to other members of that family. The most common sensitivities are to members of the Grass family which includes bamboo shoots, barley, corn, millet, oats, rye, sugar (cane), sorghum and wheat, and to the Bovid family which includes beef, veal, cheese, cream, milk, whey, yoghurt, gelatine, goat products and sheep products. Foods containing salicylates or additives and spray residues are also very important sources of sensitivity, and allergy problems such as hyperactivity.

● Rotation diet

If certain foods seem to be the cause of a sensitivity or allergic reaction, eliminate them from your diet for a while and, at the same time, also exclude other members of the family to which the suspect food belongs.

When all symptoms (the commonest are fatigue, irritability, stuffy or runny nose) are quiescent, reintroduce the suspect foods, one at a time. If there is no obvious reaction, continue to use them "in rotation", no more than once every four to five days. This will usually help you to stop building up a new sensitivity to them.

Salicylates

Among the conditions known to be caused by a salicylate sensitivity are urticaria (nettle rash), asthma, hyperactivity and some instances of colitis. How can you tell? If aspirin (active ingredient salicylic acid) makes your symptoms worse, try a low-salicylate diet. Salicylates are found in:

Aspirin tablets and medicine; many pain-killing and anti-fever preparations; teething mixtures and gripe water (read labels carefully); alfalfa (lucerne), almonds, apples, apricots, asparagus, aubergine, avocado, broad and green beans, beetroot, broccoli, carrots, chicory, courgettes, blackberries, cherries, cucumber, currants, endive, gooseberries, grapes, marrow, mushrooms, olives, onions, oranges, parsnips, peaches, peppers, plums, prunes, radishes, raisins, raspberries, spinach, strawberries, sweetcorn, tomatoes, turnips, watercress.

Condiments very high in salicylates are aniseed, cayenne, celery seed, cinnamon, dill, fenugreek, mace, mustard, oregano, paprika, rosemary, sage, thyme. Traces are found in bananas, pineapple and potato. They are found in cola drinks, tea, coffee and peppermint tea.

● Monodiets

One of the consequences of stopping eating altogether (fasting), is a rapid mobilization of effort towards elimination and detoxification. For some people this can be too rapid for comfort, and a slower version of the same detoxification process may be easier. This can best be achieved using a monodiet – a diet where only one food source such as fruit, grain or potato is eaten or drunk.

Monodiets are not only useful as general detoxification tools: they are most helpful during episodes of acute infection or, repeatedly, where there are chronic health problems, reduced vitality and general fatigue, or where there has been a history of allergy.

For anything other than short term use, you should take professional advice before fasting or monodieting, or get some degree of supervision. For a monodiet lasting 48 hours, however, you should simply avoid driving and arrange for ample rest time.

One of the odd effects of a true, water only, fast, is that after a day or so all appetite vanishes. Returning hunger is one of the signs that it is time to break a long fast. The bad news with a monodiet is that you are unlikely to lose your appetite – a disadvantage when faced with eating the same food for two whole days.

A number of monodiet variations are listed on p.83. Which should you choose?

Apple is ideal for acidic conditions such as gout or inflammation.

Grapes, especially black ones, are recommended for those with cardiac conditions; they are rich in potassium. They are marginally less effective for elimination than some other foods, but allow more energy use, so are a good choice if you have to remain active.

Citrus, such as grapefruit, is for people with liver problems or with a history of catarrh. Oranges are good for catarrh-sufferers, but can upset the liver and cause skin irritation, especially around the anus.

Those with sensitive digestions find either carrot or papaya monodiets soothing.

Rice or other cereal monodiets are effective in cases of high blood pressure.

Whichever food you choose, eat it slowly and frequently – every two hours or so. In addition drink only water, or, if on a fruit diet, the dilute juice of that fruit.

How often?
You can use a one-day monodiet as often as once a week if you wish, or need the additional detoxification. As an alternative, a weekend, or any two days at home every month to six weeks is appropriate.

Before doing a long (more than 48 hours) monodiet, you should get advice from your doctor and a nutrition expert.

Teas and juices

Your body is made of many constituent parts, but two-thirds of its weight is water, and it is important to maintain it at that level. When you lose water through sweating or other elimination channels, the concentration of minerals such as sodium in the remainder is increased. This starts a thirst cycle which prods you into drinking something to restore the correct balance.

Diets containing plenty of fruits and vegetables, which are themselves a source of water, will reduce the amount you need to drink. But unless your diet takes over 50 percent of its content from raw fruit and vegetable sources, drink not less than three pints of liquid daily – more if you perspire a lot. Pure water is still the best way to replace that lost in the elimination processes, but read the advice on p.116-17.

Herbal teas are a popular substitute for regular tea and coffee, but take care: many herb teas also contain caffeine; most contain high levels of tannin which reduces ability to absorb minerals such as iron, and some also contain specific toxic substances. Whichever you choose, try to rotate your use to reduce your chances of becoming sensitized or allergic to them.

Those known to have high levels of caffeine include Mate as well as green and black tea.

Tannin levels are high in Mate, rose-hip, yellow dock, comfrey and peppermint.

Some herbal teas (see box) have been used for centuries to ease the symptoms of common complaints. Using them in this way should never take the place of dealing with the underlying problem, however; and bear in mind that some of them are toxic if drunk in great quantities.

The safest herbal teas are lemon balm, lime flower, linden blossom, raspberry leaf, lemon grass, fennel, anise and verbena.

Special herbal teas
Elderflower for colds, flu and catarrh; red sage for similar conditions, sore throats and mouth ulcers. Thyme or peppermint for digestive upsets. Meadowsweet for diarrhoea. Chamomile relaxes and helps you sleep; eases digestive discomfort. Rosemary helps headaches and soothes digestion. Valerian for easing tension and helping sleep. For preparing for childbirth, the traditional use of raspberry leaf tea is still enormously popular.

None of these should be taken more than once or twice daily, nor for more than a few days at a time. Toxicity can result from overuse.

● Fruit juices
Why not drink fruit juice instead? The problem is the sugars. When you eat an apple, for example, the natural fruit sugars in its juice are released slowly into the bloodstream as the apple is digested. When you swallow a tumblerful of apple juice, however, sugars from the equivalent of five apples are dumped on the system all at once. This surge of sugar is controlled in your body via insulin production. No great harm arises unless you are also taking in a lot of sugary foods (again causing a rapid sugar surge) and adrenal stimulators (tea, coffee, alcohol, tobacco – and of course stress . . .), all

of which cause sugar to be released into the bloodstream, demanding yet another round of insulin production.

Medical research has shown that a rapid rise of blood sugar has an immune suppressing effect peaking two hours after consumption, making infection more likely at such a time (see p.143). Repetitive insulin surges in response to a frequent intake of rapidly absorbed forms of sugar (of any sort, whether this is brown, white, honey or fruit sugar) has been linked to damage of tissues such as the arterial walls, leading to atherosclerostic changes.

This pattern of sugar-induced troughs and highs leads to moodswings, periodic feelings of exhaustion (met by yet another sugar boost from one of the above sources) and, ultimately, adrenal and/or pancreatic failure. Hypoglycaemia and some cases of diabetes can both be traced to this pattern. So, dilute fruit juices 50:50 with water and sip them slowly; try not to exceed the amount of source fruits you would normally take; and consider the alternatives of carrot or celery juice.

Problems are compounded when you use commercially juiced products even if they do not contain added sugar; for unless it states clearly that they are organically produced, you will be getting the concentrated addition of the pesticides and fungicides off the skins. This is especially true of citrus juices, and even more so when they are concentrated.

Make your own juices, from organic produce if possible, avoiding skin if not; dilute and sip.

● Juice labels

Pay extra attention to the information on the label if you are going to drink commercially prepared fruit or vegetable juice.

Ideally the product should be organic, i.e. free of pesticide or other toxic sprays. This is less of a rarity as green consumerism spreads. Check for additives such as most preservatives, colouring or flavouring; put it back on the shelf if the word "sugar" appears. Avoid anything labelled "concentrated".

There are some safe preservatives, such as those used in a range of organic vegetable juices produced in Switzerland. These contain lactic acid which is perfectly safe and does nothing to reduce the nutrient value of the juice.

Did you know that government agencies such as the FDA in America allow a surprisingly high level of "natural and unavoidable" debris to contaminate juices . . . insects mainly?

CAUTION: anyone with a Candida problem (see p.52) should not drink fruit juices. Yeast loves sugar, and Candida is a yeast, so even fruit sugars have to be kept low while this yeast is being controlled. This means no juices, and little fruit for the first month of an anti-Candida programme.

Fasting

Fasting is the avoidance of all solid food for a period. During a fast the body uses up non-essential tissues, such as fat, as a source of fuel, but spares essential tissues. These non-essential tissues are used by the body as safe "dumping grounds" for unwanted toxic materials such as heavy metals and pesticides. When they are burned as fuel, they release the toxins which have been stored in them. This is the beginning of the detoxification process.

Fasting is not starvation, which does not begin until all non-essential tissues have been used up. This could take some weeks (or even months in some people) to begin, and you are not being asked **ever** to fast for more than 48 hours, unless under supervision.

Another important benefit from short-term fasting is that substances in your food to which you may be allergic or sensitive are temporarily avoided. For complete elimination of these allergens, though, a five-day fast is required and for this you need expert guidance.

By having a series of short fasts, combined with a generally reformed pattern of eating, drinking and living, while also using the other detoxification methods described in this book, you will safely encourage a steady detox process.

The benefits of fasting are numerous and include
*   tissue regeneration. Fasting provides a wonderful opportunity for repair and recovery in all organs and tissues. You can therefore expect your skin to look fresher and have better tone, for example, after regular fasting and detoxification.
*   energy increase. As a rule, the body becomes more efficient at producing and using energy.
*   immune function improvement (see box).
*   weight loss (likely to occur where necessary). If you did not need to lose weight, however, any lost during a fast will soon be regained as digestive and absorption functions improve afterwards.

From the detoxification point of view, periodic fasts are a major help in encouraging the necessary normalization processes.

Why a two day fast? Because it is perfectly safe. Because it fits neatly into a weekend. But chiefly because two days produces the optimum response from the immune system (see box).

It has long been known that increased resistance to infection was apparent after fasting. More recently it has been shown that during the first 35 to 48 hours of a fast, immune system functions are dramatically improved, including increased killer cell and macrophage activity, as well as cell-mediated immunity, all of which improve your defences against infectious agents such as bacteria. If a fast is longer than 48 hours, these functions go into a decline for some days – another reason for avoiding long fasts without guidance.

● Side effects of fasting

Eventually you should come to enjoy fasting for the marvel-lous sense of lightness, clarity of thought and renewed energy which it delivers. But, at first, as you start to detoxify, it may not be all that pleasant.

You can expect to have a very furred tongue and, often, a quite exceptionally unpleasant taste in your mouth on the first day of fasting. Rinse it out frequently with lemon water.

These may be accompanied by headaches and a feeling of general seediness which can be alleviated by use of the acupressure points illustrated on p.73 and the use of a coffee enema (see p.182). Do not take any medications for such symptoms as these would disrupt the fast.

Many of these symptoms are due to your body throwing out toxic debris by every means at its disposal. This is not confined to the usual channels of bowels and urine (though urine will become unusually dark), but involves the skin and mucous membranes as well.

At first your skin may look blotchy, your perspiration smelly (take extra showers or baths), and it may occur to you that the treatment is worse than the condition you are trying to improve. Be patient and see the process through: with repetition and the support of exercise, relaxation and hydrotherapy, these reactions will become less and less, and the benefits more and more obvious.

Whether the bowels function or not, use an enema once daily during a fast to ensure elimination of the accumulated debris. Other perfectly normal side-effects include feeling somewhat colder than usual (put more clothes on), and low levels of energy or ability to concentrate (rest and listen to music or the radio).

All these symptoms will pass, after the fast.

Contraindications

Do not fast
* if you are pregnant or breast feeding.
* if you are afraid of the idea; use monodiets and raw days instead. They will take longer, but eventually achieve similar results.
* if you are severely underweight or diabetic. Although both conditions can benefit from regular short fasts, these need to be supervised.
* if you have kidney or heart disease except under close supervision, ideally in an institution. Again, both conditions can benefit, but only under the right circumstances.
* if you suffer from TB.
* if you suffer from anorexia.
* if you suffer from other eating disorders – without professional supervision.

Two-day fast

On the Friday evening before a weekend fast, eat only a light salad or fruit meal, or a bowl of soup.

Saturday   You will have decided which form of fast you are following – water only, diluted juice, or potassium broth (see p.76). Have ample supplies ready and start the day with a slowly sipped half-pint tumbler of this liquid.

After dressing warmly, do your stretching exercises slowly (p.68), followed by breathing (p.63) and relaxation (p.64). Try to nap or rest during the morning, reading or listening to music or the radio.

Midmorning, or whenever you are thirsty, have another drink, and if signs of a headache appear, use the acupressure methods (p.73) to ease it.

After your lunch, another half-pint drink, try to sleep for a while. On waking, do some more stretching exercises and, if possible, have a massage (p. 71). Wash your mouth out if by now the taste is rather foul.

Weather permitting, spend half an hour outside, warmly dressed, not doing much, perhaps just walking around slowly or sitting down.

Have another drink and do your relaxation and meditation exercises before going early to bed.

Sunday   Wash your mouth out, have your breakfast drink, and do the series of stretching exercises followed by breathing and relaxation.

Whether or not the bowels work, have an enema (p.182) to cleanse the lower bowel.

Spend the morning resting, outdoors if possible, or quietly indoors. You are over half way through, now.

Continue to drink the liquid midmorning, midday and afternoon. Arrange another massage followed by a sleep.

Break your fast at around 6pm by slowly eating a stewed apple or pear, bowl of live yoghurt, or bowl of vegetable soup. You will find a little food will fill you up. Have more of the same if you are hungry later.

On Monday morning return to normal, but start with a lighter breakfast than usual.

WARNING: do not, under any circumstances, continue fasting for more than two days unless you have a health professional who both agrees that it is desirable and is also available to supervise and monitor your progress.

Wicked foods and tasty toxins

In the struggle to detoxify yourself and achieve new levels of abounding energy, it is not enough just to rid your system of the old accumulated toxins. You have to stop putting new ones in. Many undesirable foods specifically depress the immune function. These should be avoided wherever this is possible.

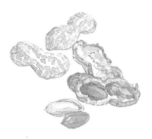

Sugar, whether white or brown (and honey too), is rapidly absorbed into the system where it suppresses the immune function and disrupts energy cycles. Our bodies need to obtain their sugar from slow release sources – vegetables, grains and proteins.

Saturated fat (from meat, dairy produce and heated oils and fats, especially those used in deep frying) is a major killer, supplying abundant opportunities for rancidity and free radical damage (see p.36) to body tissues and immune functions. (So do many flavourings, colourings and preservatives used in processed foods.)

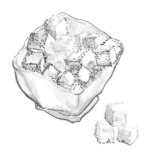

Other common hazards which are toxic and immune suppressive include:
* dried fruits (chemically processed and preserved).
* many nuts, especially peanuts, which are prone to carry highly toxic (frequently cancer-forming) moulds such as aflatoxin. Unless fresh, they can also harbour rancid oils which increase free radical damage.
* barbecued meat, which carries a mass of cancer-forming, smoke- derived toxins, as do most smoked and processed meat and fish products.
* caffeine, which is a stimulant drug plentifully found in coffee, tea, chocolate and cola drinks.

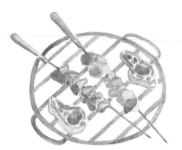

Sugar	Honey
Within 30 minutes of eating 3.5 ounces (100 grams) of sugar – any type, including honey – the bacteria-hunting and killing activity of some of your white blood cells (the neutrophil phagocytes) become depressed by up to 50 percent. This continues for up to five hours. All rapidly absorbed forms of sugar depress immune function.	As far as the immune system is concerned, honey is no different from sugar, whether white or brown. Its benefits, if the bees were not themselves fed on sugar, include traces of useful minerals, and a minute pollen content which helps hay-fever sufferers prepare their defences. Use honey sparingly on a detox diet.

Wonder foods

Just as some foods contain highly undesirable substances, so others have remarkable potential for helping to protect and detoxify us. These wonder foods are easy to find and, usually, pleasant to eat.

Garlic   This remarkable bulb contains chemicals, such as allicin, which are capable of killing most bacteria and fungi including Candida albicans. The medicinal use of garlic and its extracts is also beneficial in treating high blood pressure, intestinal parasites and many forms of toxicity. It is also able to enhance the body's capability of protecting itself against radiation damage.

Garlic also has a relatively large amount of germanium, a newly researched mineral which has been shown to enhance energy production cycles, among other useful qualities. **Caution:** avoid taking actual germanium supplements, however, as they have been shown to have toxic effect on the kidneys.

Garlic is best eaten raw: it loses some potency in cooking. Munch parsley after eating raw garlic if you find it antisocial, or just enjoy the pungent aroma and hope your friends do too, as it detoxifies your body. A number of good garlic extract capsules are now available, some of them deodorized, though the process of taking the odour out usually also takes out the beneficial effect.

Beetroot   The juice of beetroot, and therefore the uncooked vegetable itself, contains some powerful "blood-cleansing" properties. This has been much researched in Germany, Austria and Switzerland and is suggested as a useful part of detoxification. If making the juice for yourself is bothersome, organic juice, preserved with lactic acid, is generally available from health stores. Be prepared: it may turn your urine red.

Yoghurt   This virtually predigested protein food is produced when milk is cultured with either Lactobacillus bulgaricus or Streptococcus thermophilus. These bacteria do not live in the bowel, as do many other useful or some hostile bacteria. In their journey through us, however, they increase the health and wellbeing of some of the more important friendly bacteria which detoxify so much of the poison swilling through us. "Live" yoghurt is thus a major contributor to detoxification.

Yoghurt
Yoghurt is prepared from pasteurized milk using Lactobacillus bulgaricus or Streptococcus thermophilus. If it is again pasteurized, i.e. after the culture has developed (often done to extend its shelf-life), the bacteria are killed, making the yoghurt dead and therefore useless for detoxification purposes, though still a useful source of protein.

Whether you choose cows' or goats', insist on yoghurt with "live" or "unpasteurized" on its carton, or learn how to make your own.

Adaptogens

Some rare foods and substances are able to help the body adapt more successfully to stress of any sort. These adaptogens offer general rather than specific benefits, so it is important they should be free of unexpected side effects.

By definition, adaptogens seem to produce a number of benefits to various body functions, protecting against a variety of stress factors. They influence the body's self-repairing, self-balancing mechanisms, allowing them to operate more efficiently, whatever form of adaptation is being called for.

Most adaptogens have a long history of use as folk remedies and are now well researched, especially when urgent new needs arise such as the need to protect cosmonauts from radiation damage (see box).

In a detoxification programme their value lies in the way they can assist the smooth alterations in function needed as your body deals with the elimination of toxic debris and the regeneration of organs and tissues.

Because of the enormous popularity of adaptogens, ginseng and royal jelly in particular, some dubious products have appeared on the market. It pays to ask for expert advice and try to get genuine products from health stores.

Doses
You may wish to take one of these adaptogens for general protection during detoxification or stress. Doses suggested are: Eleutherococcus or ginseng: half to one gram daily; or Royal jelly: 1-2 generous teaspoonsful daily; or Pollen: 1-5 grams (usually capsules or tablets) daily.

Cosmonauts
Over 20,000 substances were studied by Russian scientists searching for ways to reduce the damage produced by radiation exposure in their space programme. Only a few were consistently effective, including two related plant products, ginseng and its cousin, Siberian eleutherococcus. Both have folk lore traditions going back centuries, and both are now known for their safe, multiple protective health benefits.

Siberian eleutherococcus
In studies both this, and/or oriental ginseng, protected animal tissue from the effects of radiation. Radiation damage results from chain reactions of cell destruction due to highly charged free radical substances (see p. 36); this is the same way most toxic materials harm you. Use of such adaptogens, in tablet or tea form, reduces toxic damage.

Royal jelly
This food, produced by worker bees to feed their queen, is a powerful adaptogen. It contains very high proportions of specific nutrients, notably vitamin B5. The life span of experimental animals of all sorts is increased significantly by royal jelly, even when they are exposed to a variety of toxic and stress factors.

Pollen
Pollen extracts consist of a highly nutritious mix of substances including essential fatty acids and vitamins. They seem to act in ways very similar to those of royal jelly.

Supplements

Surveys of apparently healthy people of all ages by reputable health authorities, throughout Europe and the US, prove that most people show evidence of at least one, and sometimes many, deficiencies of the 50 or so vitamins or minerals known to be essential for health.

This is both because of the sort of food chosen and because of the decline in the nutrient content of many foods, due to methods of production, manufacture and storage. For example, food irradiation destroys massive amounts of vitamin content in the quest for improved shelf-life (especially antioxidants such as vitamin E).

Added to this, we all have our own unique nutritional requirements. These are partly related to our in-born idiosyncrasies (biochemical individuality) and partly to needs related to our age, occupation, stress and toxin exposure, state of health, and ability to absorb nourishment readily.

This combination of poor raw materials and specific needs suggests that some supplementation of nutritional factors would be sound insurance. This is all the more sensible when you are coping with detoxification, and the processes of adaptation as you move towards a higher level of health.

When multivitamin/mineral supplements are taken as a "health insurance", there is absolutely no danger of side-effects and a very real chance of assisting general function – and the cost of such a strategy is not high.

Specific nutritional support may be indicated by your scores in some of the questionnaires, over and above general supplementation suggested during the detoxification programmes.

Medical students and biochemical individuality

Professor Roger Williams' work at Texas University resulted in the understanding that our needs for each and every vitamin, mineral and amino acid are quite unique.

From among his own students he showed that, in any group of ten or fifteen, all in apparently perfect health, some would have biochemical needs for a nutrient – any nutrient – which varied a great deal from others in the group; and he seldom found any two students who had exactly the same requirements. One might need five, ten or fifteen times the vitamin C, calcium or any other nutrient to stay in good health than another. If these students were all eating the same sort of food it was not surprising that some were not giving their bodies what they needed.

This is true of all of us: levels recommended by government agencies are just averages, and none of us is average in everything.

Supplements. Do –

* Take only recommended dosages; because some is good, more is not necessarily better.
* Take all suggested supplements with or after meals, except when specifically told otherwise.
* Take all fat-soluble supplements (vitamins A, K, E and essential fatty acids) with a meal containing some oils or fats, for better absorption.
* Take any amino acid supplements away from meals and away from protein drinks e.g. milk; this would retard its absorption. Absorption is usually improved, however, by taking amino acids just after a very small amount of carbohydrate such as a mouthful of bread.
* Store supplements in a cool dark place.
* Look carefully at label for expiry date and any special instructions about storage, such as refrigeration.
* If zinc needs to be supplemented, take it last thing at night; it is better absorbed then.
* Take any supplements regularly and for a lengthy period; some take months to be absorbed in any useful quantity.
* Try to get natural, organic, sources of vitamins rather than synthetic, inorganic ones. This is not always easy.
* Look carefully at labels, avoiding any which contain unnecessary additives. All tablets have to be held together by something; make sure it is safe for you.
* Use powdered forms if you cannot find safe tablets.
* Look for the words "hypoallergenic" or "free from common allergens". If you have allergies, the label should ideally state, "Contains no lactose, yeast, starch, sugars, gluten or preservatives". "Yeast and sugar free" are especially important for Candida problems.

Supplements: Don'ts

* Don't take vitamin E at the same time as iron supplements (if both are needed); separate intake by at least ten hours.
* Don't take the entire dose of any water-soluble vitamin (C and the B complex group) in one go; split the dose up and spread intake through the day.
* Don't ever take more selenium or vitamin B6 than recommended. They are extremely useful in normal doses but can cause toxic reactions if overdone.
* Don't be alarmed if, when you are taking high doses of vitamin C, you develop diarrhoea. This normal, harmless sign that you are taking too much will cease when you cut back.
* Don't take supplements (apart from multivitamin and/or multiminerals) if you are pregnant without clear advice from your physician.
* Don't take any single B vitamin (B1, 2, 3, 5, 6 or 12) for any time without also supplementing, at another time on the same day, the entire B-complex, as imbalance can otherwise easily develop.
* Don't eat raw egg whites; they stop absorption of Biotin, one of the B- vitamins.
* Don't assume that supplements can't harm you if you are already taking prescription medication. Diabetics and heart patients, particularly, could find that vitamin C and E supplements necessitate a lower dose of their medication. Always consult your doctor or health professional,
* Don't take high doses of vitamin E if you have high blood pressure; start with low doses and gradually increase.
* Don't be alarmed if your urine turns green or dark yellow when B vitamins are supplemented; this is normal.
* Don't take shiny tablets unless they state "sugar free".

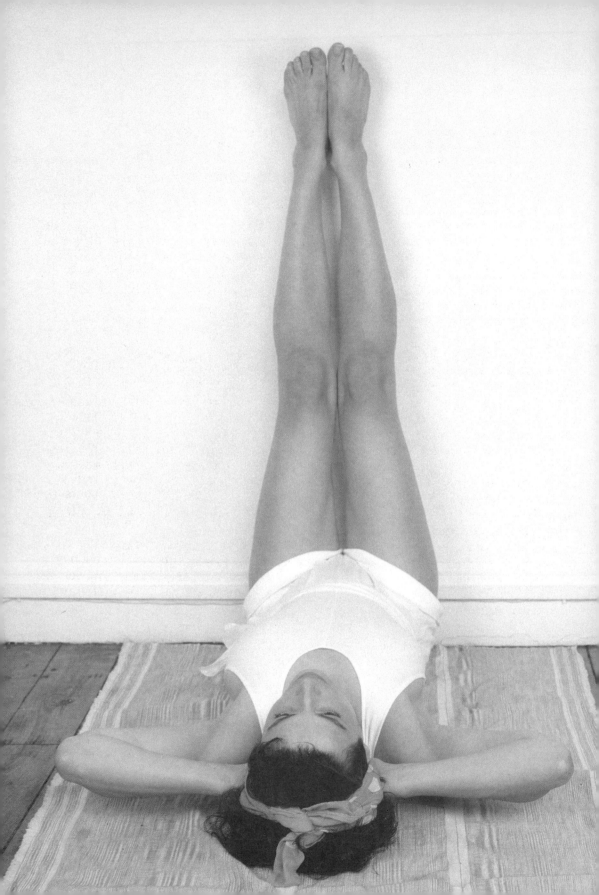

Exercise and breathing

You can secure improvements in many bodily functions, especially breathing and circulation, from regular aerobic exercise.

As part of a detoxification programme the achievement of such improvements is absolutely fundamental. Adequate regular exercise improves elimination through the skin, encourages greater detoxification through the lungs, better oxygenation and repair of tissues and organs, and enhanced overall circulation and heart function. Additionally, exercise stimulates greater energy production, and your metabolic rate – the speed at which your basic functions operate – accelerates as well, to the great benefit of overall detoxification levels.

Aerobic exercise also stimulates the release in the brain of natural hormones called beta endorphins. These compounds produce a feeling of happiness, even euphoria – and you don't have to run a marathon to experience this. Indeed, people using static exercise cycles are able to achieve this "rush", commonly known as "jogger's high".

This biochemical transformation is far more significant than just a good feeling, though; it is evidence of a major body-method for dealing with stress. Walking, jogging, cycling or skipping are all stress reducers, as well as health enhancers. They are also ways of achieving "active meditation". As you perform the repetitive physical motions involved, you focus on the mechanics of what you are doing; when you achieve this to the exclusion of outside thoughts you are, in effect, meditating (see p.107) and gaining the mental and physical benefits of that meditative state.

To be really beneficial, aerobic exercise has to be done properly. This means a minimum of at least enough exercise, done three times a week on alternate days, to produce the aerobic effect for the duration of thirty minutes.

The degree of exercise needed to achieve this effect is almost certainly different in you from that required in someone else; for part of the beauty of this marvellous system is that it is tailored to your individuality, as measured by your resting pulse and your age (see p.70). Only when you have carefully worked out the formula that gives you your two pulse rate markers, below the first of which you are achieving little, and above the second of which you are doing too much and straining yourself, can you begin to achieve aerobic effects and benefits.

You will find that as you get fitter, you need to do more and more to get your pulse rate up to the right level: evidence absolute of your increasing fitness. Your respiratory function, important for long-term health maintenance, will also improve.

Mental health improves with physical health, so you will find greater peace of mind, better powers of concentration and higher levels of arousal as your body responds. The ability of your body to deal with toxicity will become more highly developed, and this will give you a better chance of lasting standards of high-level wellbeing.

Choosing your exercise

There is a great deal more to exercising than meets the eye at first. For the legions of the unfit, it may seem enough to perform any activity outside the normal sedentary routine that gets you out of breath and, perhaps, pleasantly achey. However, a more serious attempt at assessment will address the need to balance considerations of pleasure and safety with the availability of facilities and, most important, whether the exercise you choose will deliver the goods — whether it will be effective. This calls for some planning.

Your objective is clear: to improve the cardiovascular function, to encourage a greater and more efficient use of oxygen, with consequent increases in excretion of wastes through the lungs and skin. Overall, you are looking for a permanent increase in metabolic rate, even during the time you are not exercising.

The aerobic system, which was developed by Dr Kenneth Cooper, has been adopted by both the US and Royal Canadian Air Forces as their major fitness programme. It uses normal activity to improve overall health via its revolutionary methodology and allows you to test yourself, decide how much activity you actually require, and even to measure your own progress. Most people who use this method find a great increase in wellbeing, with many minor health symptoms vanishing. This is due to a combination of enhanced cardiovascular/circulatory function, improved detoxification, and stress reduction, all associated with a more normal metabolic rate.

Any form of exercise which increases the body's ability to deliver oxygen-bearing blood to the muscles and organs is "aerobic". The chief disadvantage of some forms of exercise is that they are not aerobic. The periods of rest involved in such "anaerobic" activities as squash, tennis, volleyball or basketball, for example, interrupt the aerobic effect by allowing the heart to slow down. Swimming, otherwise such a wonderful general muscle toner, certainly can be a good aerobic conditioner but only achieves aerobic levels if you do it over an extended period of time; and weight training is never going to help in an aerobic sense as it involves mainly static activity. All these are excellent for their own purposes although they fall short in terms of our particular goal; any regular exercise keeps the metabolic rate at a high normal level, develops the body's lean tissues, uses up fat, and helps adjust your appetite-control level.

Try to find aerobic activities which give you pleasure. Joining an aerobic class can bring you companionship,

CAUTION: if you scored high in the hypoglycaemia, diabetes or cardiovascular questionnaires (p.52-3), or are chronically tired, do not do any aerobic exercise until you have your doctor's all clear. If you have joint problems, with your back or hips for instance, which preclude some of the more jarring exercises, think about swimming, static cycling and walking as the safer choices.

discipline, encouragement and the reassurance that you are using your efforts to best advantage. Look for classes with properly qualified and trained staff, where the emphasis is on safety.

Cycling is another choice. Advantages are that it can either be combined with travel or done safely at home on a static exercise cycle. Of all the options available, cycling combines the lowest risk of damage to the various parts of the body (aside from the perils associated with being out in traffic) with being extremely effective.

Jogging and running give excellent aerobic results but you need soft going on which to do them. Be sure that there is nothing wrong with any of your weight-bearing joints such as knees or hips, since pounding hard pavements is one of the best ways of damaging them in the long term.

Skipping and aerobic dancing are ideal indoor activities and appeal to many people but, again, problems with weight-bearing joints, or the back, can rule them out.

There are some rules you should not break: the first is do NOT skip the essential warm-up exercises described on p.156. You must make yourself do these before any aerobic session to avoid injuring yourself.

Next, you must have the right equipment. Running and walking demand the best training shoes and an appropriate track suit. Skipping and dancing require a suitable floor covering so you avoid jarring yourself on a hard surface. Aerobics should be fun and not a chore, but it is up to you to make it safe.

Above all, do aerobic exercise regularly: not less than every other day, and for between 20 and 30 minutes. During this time your pulse rate must be raised above the lower of the two measurements calculated (p.70) and not higher than the second.

The Basic programme of stretching and exercise (p.68–70) will already have helped you achieve an improvement in your resting morning pulse rate, and this is a good point at which to reassess your safe aerobic levels.

Keep a record of what you achieve from now on, not only rechecking your pulse levels every few months but also seeing just how you are doing as you get fitter. How long did you take to walk (jog, cycle or swim) a mile or two miles when you began? How long does it take you now? How many continuous skips could you do at the start – 100, 150, more? How many now? Give yourself targets; enjoy aerobics; and take pride in the results.

High stress scorers' advice

If you scored high in the stress questionnaire on p.47 you should take your introduction to aerobics slowly. The exercises demand adaptation from your body, and this is a form of stress in itself. So don't be in a hurry; concentrate more time on the warm-up processes and do only a ten minute aerobic activity three times a week at first. After a few weeks extend this by a few minutes each time until, after several months, you are doing the full 30 minutes on alternate days.

Breathing

Correct breathing is vital to wellbeing. The introductory exercises on p.63 will have helped you to focus on this, but before going further you must make sure that the machinery with which you breathe is able to do its job. Any areas of muscular restriction between your ribs, for example, will severely limit their ability to open and close freely as part of normal breathing.

Pay attention to the way you breathe. You may be using only a part of the respiratory capacity available to you. Many factors including posture (round shoulders or a ramrod bearing are equally bad), work and other daily habits have an effect on the structure of the body and influence breathing. Emotional stress and habits such as smoking have obvious negative effects, preventing full and free expansion of the chest.

As you sit quietly, or walk about, or apply yourself to work and play, observe the patterns of your breathing cycle. Try to feel where in your body you breathe. In the upper chest? Or down in the abdomen? Where do you feel restricted when you are breathing heavily?

These exercises will help you release such restrictions and normalize breathing. When you breathe properly, you can eliminate the toxins which the body should be removing via this route most effectively, and allow adequate oxygenation of the blood, so increasing energy.

The exercise on this page uses bending of the body to open out the rib cage. It stretches the small muscles between the ribs, increases their range of motion and lets you practise breathing into these opened-up regions. Do this for a few days before moving to the exercises described opposite.

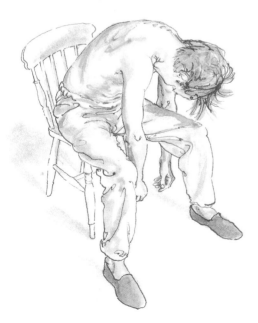

With left arm between knees and right outside, turn head to the right and breathe slowly and deeply into your upper right back so you feel the muscles stretch. Hold breath for 5-10 seconds and, as you slowly release it, stretch hands towards floor, opening the area even more. Repeat five times. Turn head to the other side, change arm positions and repeat process. By varying the degree and angle of your "bend", you can focus on different areas, covering most of the upper rib structures.

CAUTION: sit quietly for a minute before getting up or you may feel dizzy.

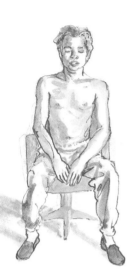

Sit in front of a mirror and breathe deeply. If your shoulders rise, you are mistakenly using upper shoulder and neck muscles for breathing. To correct this, sit in an upright chair with arms. Press elbows down firmly on the arms as you inhale; this holds your shoulders down. Breathe deeply, in and out, for three minutes twice daily.

2. Rest hands on lower ribs and breathe in deeply (3-4 seconds) so hands are pushed apart sideways. As you breathe out (4-5 seconds) push slightly towards centre to encourage complete exhalation. Repeat 15 times.

Full breathing cycle

1. Lie on floor, pillow under knees; rest hands on abdomen above navel. Breathe in deeply (3-4 seconds) so hands are lifted slightly towards ceiling. As you breathe out (4-5 seconds) apply light pressure towards floor to encourage complete exhalation. Repeat 15 times.

3. Rest hands on upper chest. Breathe in deeply (3-4 seconds) so you feel hands rising slightly towards ceiling. As you breathe out (4-5 seconds) apply slight pressure towards floor, ensuring complete exhalation. Repeat 15 times.

Experience the sequence of abdomen rising, lower chest expanding sideways, upper chest filling and rising; followed by upper chest falling, lower chest coming together and abdomen falling: a normal breathing cycle. Rest quietly after such exercise to avoid dizziness.

Stretching

Yoga stretching postures (asanas) are uniquely gentle yet effective ways of making your body healthier, more supple and more pliable. The combination of breathing and unhurried isometric stretches distinguishes yoga from other methods of stretching, and enables you to achieve the state of mental calm which is its characteristic.

It is important to combine such forms of stretching with exercise of a more active kind, such as aerobics, to avoid the development of over-toned musculature. This (see p.68) both wastes energy and retards lymphatic circulation and drainage – fundamental aspects of detoxification.

The principles of yoga demand that you always do its exercises slowly. Never force yourself to the limit of motion in any particular direction, nor to the point of pain. Just take the feeling that you are stretching strongly as far as is comfortable. Breathe deeply and slowly as you hold a posture, ideally for about a minute before, **on a strong exhalation**, taking yourself a little further into the direction of stretch. Hold this for another minute as you breathe deeply and relax before coming slowly out of one posture and adopting the next.

The sequences illustrated on these pages combine to stretch and relax most of the important postural muscles of the body – the group which has the greatest tendency to tighten through abuse or lack of use. Do not start them, however, until you have been doing the exercises on p.68 for some weeks; then do them at least every other day.

Follow the guidelines: the mild stretch asked for should stop short of any pain.

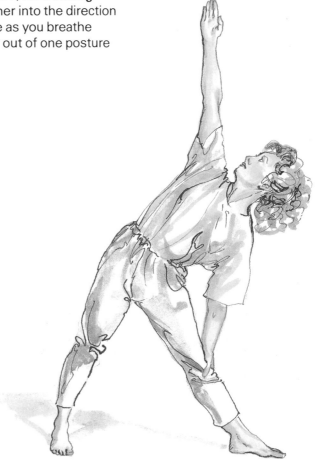

The Triangle effectively stretches all the muscles on the side of the body from the foot to the neck. Stand, legs a yard apart, with left foot turned left and right foot slightly left. Extend arms sideways at shoulder level, palms downwards. On breathing out, bend sideways from the hips, taking your left arm down to grasp your left leg, while your other arm goes up towards the ceiling. Turn your head to look up at your thumb. Make sure you are not bending forward or backwards, but purely sideways. Tighten the muscles to lift and stretch the knees and stretch your arms to their comfortable maximum range. After about a minute of slow breathing in this posture, exhale strongly and ease a little more into the direction of stretch. Hold this for another minute before coming back up to the starting position. Reverse all positions to stretch the other side.

The Plough stretches all the spinal and some of the leg and neck muscles. Inverting the digestive organs improves circulation and drainage functions, so even if your feet do not reach the floor behind your head in the full yoga posture illustrated, take them over the head and backwards, letting them dangle there.

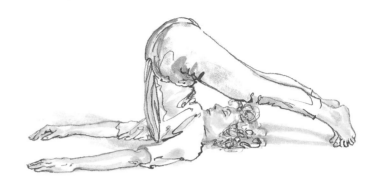

Lie on back on floor, arms at sides; breathe in. Bend both knees on to the abdomen, then straighten them up, supporting lower back with hands. Exhale, taking legs over head; hold for a minute before slowly returning to flat position.

The Warrior position stretches shoulder and upper chest muscles. Stretch one hand up behind your back and try to grasp other hand which has been taken forwards, over and backwards. Stay at point of maximum stretch for a minute and breathe slowly. On exhalation, increase the stretch on both arms. Stay in this position another minute then slowly change over to the opposite direction.

The Half Spinal Twist releases tensions in the small rotator muscles of the back. Anyone with a history of back problems should use it carefully. It has beneficial effects on the internal organs as it gently compresses them.

Kneel on the floor, legs tucked together, buttocks on heels. Bring right leg forward and cross it over the other so the right foot rests with its heel close to left buttock. Keep

your back straight. Grasp right foot or left knee with left hand. As you breathe out, twist around to the right, resting your right hand on the floor behind your body. Hold, breathing slowly, for at least a minute before, on exhalation, twisting and turning a little further. Hold for another minute before slowly coming back to the original position. Do everything in reverse.

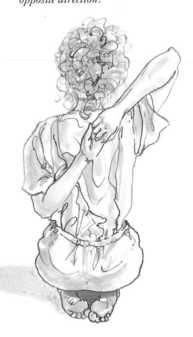

Warm-up stretches

Do warm-up exercises before any vigorous aerobic prog-ramme to prevent injury or strain (see p.151). The other stretching and yoga exercises (p.68-9, 104-5, and 154-5) also bring you increased mobility and suppleness. These stretches effectively flush the muscles with freshly oxygen-ated blood and release local tensions, making them far less likely to become strained. As well as going through these warm-up stretches before aerobic activity, you can do them any time you feel stiffness or tightness developing in particular muscles.

CAUTION: use only light stretching for safety. Con-sult your doctor if you have a history of neck problems.

These exercises work on the "muscle-energy" principles explained on p.104-5 and should always be performed slowly, taking the muscles in question to a strong, but never painful, degree of stretch. Hold this for ten seconds before, on release of a breath, the isometric effect allows the muscle to release, giving an increased degree of stretch.

Hamstring stretch

Hamstrings are a group of mus-cles which run behind the thigh from the upper leg to below the knee. They are among those muscles most likely to be in-jured during unaccustomed ex-ercise. They are major postural muscles and therefore have a tendency to shorten when over or under used. By stretching them before exercise you great-ly reduce the risk of injury. This stretch, or a variation of it, is one you will see sprinters performing with great dedica-tion before any competition.

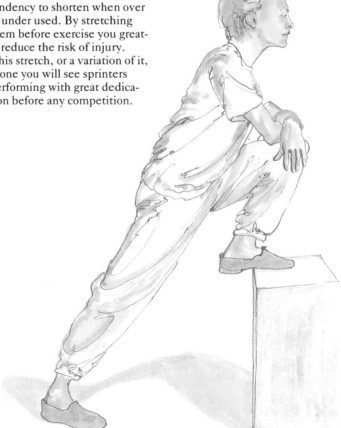

Stand in front of a chair or box. Place the leg to be stretched half a pace behind you and the other flat on the box so that the toes and ball of the foot are resting on it. Rest your folded arms on your front knee and, keeping the back straight all the time, *bend the front knee and lean forwards until you feel a strong, but not painful, degree of stretch in the back of the straight leg. Hold for ten seconds and then, as you release your breath, lean – don't bend – for-ward a little more, slightly increas-ing the stretch. Hold for another ten seconds and then change legs.*

The pectoral muscles run from your chest to your upper arms. If they are short, they can be injured easily during active exercise, and need stretching. *The trapezius*, lying between your shoulder and neck, is commonly involved in neck tension and headache problems. *The sternomastoid* runs down the front (side) of the neck; it is involved in all neck movements and is a major cause of head and neck problems when tight.

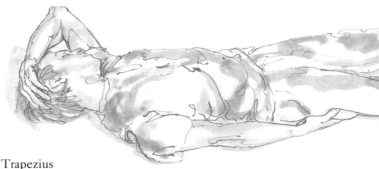

Trapezius
Lie on the floor with left hand under left buttock. Take right hand over your head, pulling away from the shoulder thus "fixed" to the point of maximum comfortable stretch. Breathe in and gently try to bring the "fixed" left shoulder up towards the left ear, and the ear down towards the shoulder, resist-ing both movements (by lying on the arm and holding the head firmly). After ten seconds stop the effort and ease the head a little further away from the shoulder, stretching the muscle between them slightly. Now do the other side.

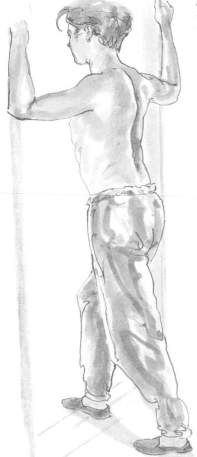

Doorway stretch for pectoral muscles
Stand in a doorway, upper arms parallel with the floor, hands grasping the frame. Place one leg behind you and, keeping the trunk straight all the time, lean the upper body forwards, placing a stretching strain on the muscles on the front of the upper chest and upper arms. Hold for ten seconds and, as you release a breath, lean further forwards, increasing the stretch slightly. Hold for another ten seconds and release.

Sternomastoid
Lie face-up on a bed with your head just over the edge, turned away from the side to be stretched; rest your hand on the forehead. Gently try to lift the head as you resist the effort with your hand. Hold for ten seconds and then release, allowing gravity to stretch the muscle for 20 seconds. Turn to the other side and stretch the muscle on the other side of the neck.

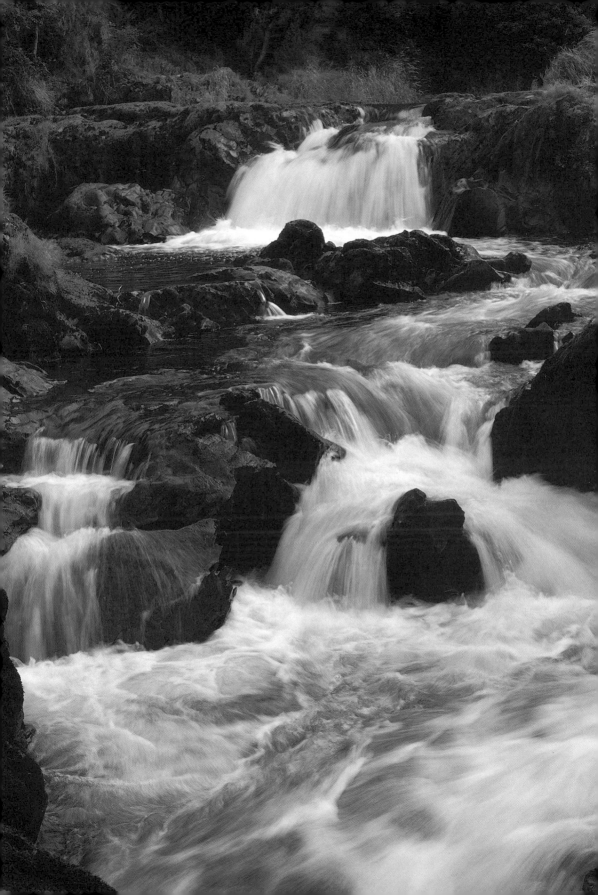

Water therapies

The water therapies used in these pro-grammes are just a few of the hundreds available to traditional hydrotherapy both as originally practised in Germany and Austria by healer/priests in the last century, and as still used throughout Europe and the US in spas and clinics today. The variations we have chosen are relatively easy and in-expensive to use at home, and they specifi-cally assist in detoxification through the skin. As a bonus, some bring major rela-xation benefits; you will find you experi-ence levels of profound relaxation over and above the stress release achieved through specific exercise patterns (p.102) and medi-tation (p.107). And almost all have benefi-cial effects on circulation functions (try the skin brushing technique on p.66 for imme-diate results). Further, you can expect skin related conditions to improve, local circu-lation to be enhanced with consequent improvements in skin tone and colour, and chronic catarrhal problems to disappear as toxic debris is excreted through the skin rather than through the mucous mem-branes. The better the eliminative functions through the skin, of course, the less stress is placed on the other organs working on this job – the lungs, kidneys and bowels.

When you sweat, moisture passes through the skin. While the primary pur-pose of sweating is to keep you cool when you are hot (the moisture cools you as it evaporates), debris gets washed away on this tide of fluid elimination. The more effi-cient the circulation to and from your skin, and the better equipped your pores for allowing sweat through, the more debris you will be able to eliminate.

Water treatments encourage these func-tions in various ways, each working on a particular part of the mechanism. Some methods will increase general circulation to bring more debris to the skin's surface for elimination, while others encourage the healthy status of the skin itself, ensuring that layers of dead tissue are actively removed, and the channels left clear.

Other water therapy techniques are designed specifically to improve circulation in the digestive areas and the pelvis. These improve the digestive function and – most important – the detoxifying capability of the liver. The Sitz bath (p.164), for example, tones the internal abdominal organs and helps to "flush" along sluggish movement of fluid which would otherwise slow down the detoxification processes. Few hydro-therapy methods have such marvellous, almost instantaneous, effect; its drawback lies in the somewhat complicated mech-anics of having to organise hot and cold water containers for rapid alternation of temperature.

This chapter introduces you to some of the ways in which hydrotherapy furthers these aims. As you become more aware of them, try to incorporate into your detoxifi-cation and stress reducing programme those methods which suit you best. Try them all, at least a few times each, before selecting those which make you feel good and which are least trouble to organise. Have fun with them.

The principles of hydrotherapy

Hydrotherapy harnesses some of the physical properties of water – its ability to retain heat and cold, for example – to the porous nature of the skin for the performance of certain functions which have a helpfully detoxifying effect.

In the setting of the home we are a bit limited by lack of space and the specialist equipment that might be found in clinics or spas, but much can stiill be done. For example, the whole body or trunk pack (p.160) uses only commonly available materials. When a pack is first applied, the damp, cool material rapidly absorbs heat from your body. The insulating layer retains this heat, with several desirable consequences: it improves local circulation, it has pro-foundly relaxing effects on muscles, and the profuse sweating results in impressive elimination through the skin. Evidence of this elimination is to be found when the pack materials are washed out later; they will have become discoloured and highly acidic.

Sitz baths (p.164) have similar short term effects on pelvic (and therefore digestive) functions as do trunk packs. They exploit another combination of water- and body-properties to improve circulation: the effect on the body of dunking it alternately in hot and cold water is to achieve a rapid circulatory interchange which "flushes" the region with new oxygenated blood. This moves stagnant fluids smartly on.

Perhaps the symbiosis of skin and water is at its most pleasing when various herbal and other ingredients (p.162-3) are added to ordinary baths. Herbs absorbed inwards through the skin allow their particular properties to influence detoxification; while other substances such as clay increase elimination out through the skin. Both approaches, used diligently, improve the body's detoxification processes.

Rub salt on your skin (p.161) to clear it of debris and to stimulate – just try it and see! – circulation of blood to the surface, dredging up its burden of toxic waste for elimination. It is a good idea to vary the hydrotherapy methods you use as constant repetition of the same method (say, daily salt glow or sitz bath) reduces the efficiency of your body's response to it.

The beauty of hydrotherapy lies in its simplicity and effectiveness if the guiding rules are carefully followed.

CAUTION: never use hyd-rotherapy methods soon after mealtimes. Allow one hour to elapse.

Don't use very hot or very cold water applications if you have kidney or car-diovascular conditions without first checking with your doctor. Although prob-lems with these organs do not altogether rule out hyd-rotherapy, there is a chance that you could impose an undue strain on yourself when applying self- treatment.

Salt glow

Salt glow stimulates the skin and its use will be helpful for people who have difficulty sweating or who have poor circulation to hands and feet, or who have a chronic rheumatic-type history. Diabetics who use insulin, people with serious cardiovascular disease or people with open or weeping skin rashes should avoid using it.

Sit on a stool in the shower or bath. Put half a cup of coarse salt (table salt will do but coarse is better) in a quart-sized bowl; moisten it just enough to make the grains stick together. Take a tablespoonful onto each hand and friction it onto the skin of one leg, starting near the foot and working briskly upwards. Take more salt as you need it and cover the whole leg. Do the same with the other leg, then one arm and then the other. Next friction as much of your back as you can reach (if a partner or friend can do all this for you so much the better) and, finally, your abdomen and chest, avoiding breast tissue.

After the full salt friction, rinse off using a shower or hand shower and warm but not hot water. Rub the skin with your hands as the water rinses the salt off and use a vigorous motion with the towel as you dry.

Go straight to bed. Make sure that there are no draughts and that you are well covered. You should sleep very deeply and may perspire profusely. This effect will become less obvious as skin health improves and detoxification progresses. At the start of a detox programme it is an extremely useful method.

How often?
Use a salt glow once a week if you have difficulty in sweating. If not, do it at least once a month during the detoxification programme, or now and again as the fancy takes you.

Sit on a stool in the shower. Before letting the water run, rub moistened salt vigorously onto each leg, each arm and back, abdomen and chest. Use up- and-down or circular movements and try to obtain a good deal of friction. Rinse well with warm water and towel dry.

Baths

Submerging your body in water is an excellent way to detoxify since it allows substances in the water to influence the entire body surface, excluding the head. Essential oils, oatmeal, peat and clay can all be used in this way with beneficial results.

Essential oils are derived from the odoriferous part of plants. They have physiological effects on the body and can influence blood pressure, stimulate nerve function, and aid digestion. Shake a few drops of oil, chosen from those listed below, onto the surface of the bath water and swish it to disperse them (too great a concentration would irritate the skin). As you enter, your body will pick up a fine coating of the oil. Now lie back, and relax, absorbing it through your skin, and breathing in the gentle vapours as the essence slowly evaporates in the heat of the water.

You may prefer to apply essential oils directly onto the skin. After a bath or shower, when the hot water has opened the pores, pour a few drops into the palm of your hand and massage it in gently so the oil reaches and penetrates down through the skin.

An oatmeal bath is recommended for anyone who finds that the detox programme is making their skin irritated or itchy, or who has a tendency to eczema or hives. Such local irritation is usually due to the rapid elimination through the skin of toxic, acidic wastes. Oatmeal is very soothing, but you will also need to take extra care over regular washing, and the changing of underclothes and bedding.

Oatmeal bath
Tie one pound of uncooked oatmeal in a large piece of gauze. Hang or hold this under the hot tap so the water runs through, encouraging the release of its essential ingredients. Float bag in water or use it as a 'sponge', rubbing your skin with it. Alternatively, grind large cup of rolled oats in a processor and stir into bath.

Stay in the water at 96°C for at least 20 minutes to give irritated skin maximum benefit. Pat – don't rub – yourself dry.

Essential oils
Buy pure, essential oils from herb shops, health stores or body shops. Those listed here have a profound effect on detoxification, according to your choice.

Cedarwood: antiseptic, sedative and promotes elimination through mucous membranes.

Chamomile: calming, pain relieving, antibacterial and digestive aid.

Juniper: increases urine flow, digestive stimulant, tonic.

Lemon: increases urine flow, tonic, antiseptic.

Olibaum: encourages sweating.

Rose: stimulates liver, stomach functions, anti-depressant effect.

Tea-tree: antifungal, antibiotic, skin function enhancer.

How often?
The oatmeal bath can be taken as often as you like to soothe itchiness if and whenever it happens. Take it at any time of the day.

Essential oil baths should, ideally, be taken last thing at night and, in any case, well away from mealtimes. Use them several times a week if you find them pleasant and helpful.

Peat baths

Peat consists of compacted decaying leaves, roots and mosses. It contains resin, silica, sulphur, carbonic iron, a variety of salts and non-harmful levels of acids such as sulphuric acid. These micro-elements in peat can be absorbed through the skin and used with benefit in many conditions including rheumatic and skin problems. Its semi-fluid state makes possible the transfer through the skin of a remarkable number of useful chemical substances, and this quality can be useful for neutralizing toxic substances on and under the skin.

Among peat's medically recorded attributes is evidence of its lowering high blood pressure, reducing high blood sugar levels, improving local circulation, solving problems of excessive acidity, and increasing alkaline mineral reserves in the body. Peat has the remarkable quality of seeming cooler than it really is, so allowing comfortable application to the skin at temperatures which, related to water, would feel unacceptably high.

Ideally peat should be mixed into a soft paste and spread quite thickly onto as much of the body surface as possible. In the home setting this is not really a serious proposition due to the incredible messiness of the whole procedure. A bath, using a liquid peat extract from the pharmacy, is a more sensible alternative. Peat is found naturally in most countries, but some of the best liquid extracts are Austrian.

Simply pour the appropriate amount of liquid peat extract (follow instructions on the container) into a hot bath (around 98°C) and soak for a good 20 minutes. Afterwards shower and get into a warm bed. Be prepared to sweat.

Another naturally-occurring substance, clay, is a useful detoxifying medium. Sometimes called "Bentonite", it is a unique kind of earth: it is almost impermeable, wet or dry; and it has long been used in folk medicine as a means of "drawing out" impurities and toxicities from the body when applied in the form of a poultice. Taken internally, dissolved in water, or as a pellet, it attracts toxic material to itself while passing through the digestive tract.

Used externally, French green clay, in particular, has remarkable qualities of neutralising toxic substances, as well as of being able to draw these through the skin. While peat adds vital detoxifying substances to the body, clay draw toxins out. Although their ways of working differ somewhat, both achieve similar end results.

Other baths
Add a pound of French green clay to a hot (98°C) bath, dissolving it completely so that it can come into contact with the whole body. Or, alternatively, moisten clay into a paste and plaster it over large or local areas of the body. Leave it in place for an hour or so before showering or bathing it off.

Sitz bath

This traditional German/Austrian hydrotherapeutic method has a stimulating effect on the circulation. Most "Kurhauses" (spas) in Germany and elsewhere in Europe still use this method extensively.

For greatest effect you need two containers. Ideally you would use the old-fashioned hip-bath, but large plastic bowls may have to do. They must be big enough to sit in with some room to spare. Half fill one with hot — not boiling — water, and the other with cold — the colder the better. Two further containers are required, one for cold water and the other for hot. While you are sitting up to your navel in hot water, your feet will be in cold; and, vice versa, when you are sitting in cold, your feet will be in hot water.

If you cannot find enough suitable containers to take the sitz bath as described, run hot water into your bathtub and place in it a bowl of cold water big enough for your feet. After the prescribed length of time, get out, let the water out, run cold water and place in it a foot container of hot water. The delay between hot and cold immersion, unfortunately, means that it cannot be as effective as it should be, but it would be better than nothing.

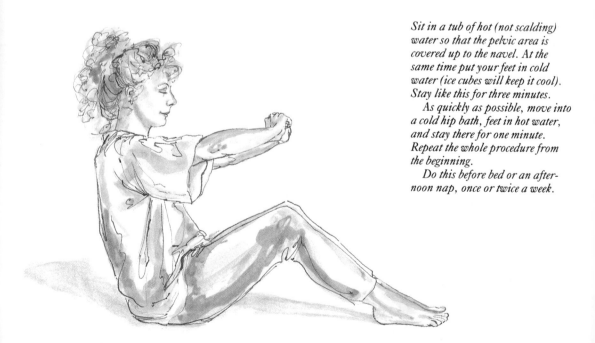

Sit in a tub of hot (not scalding) water so that the pelvic area is covered up to the navel. At the same time put your feet in cold water (ice cubes will keep it cool). Stay like this for three minutes.

As quickly as possible, move into a cold hip bath, feet in hot water, and stay there for one minute. Repeat the whole procedure from the beginning.

Do this before bed or an afternoon nap, once or twice a week.

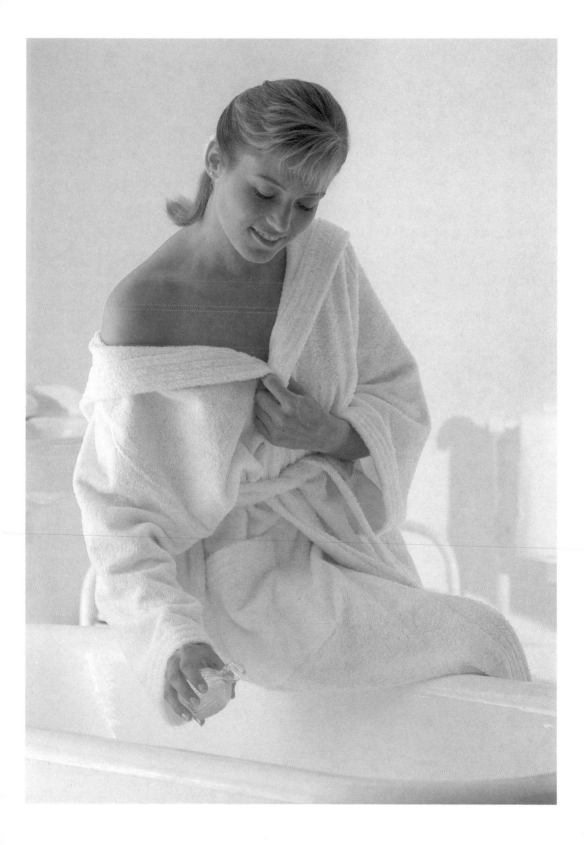

Packs, saunas and Epsom salts

Packs and saunas work by increasing sweating and hence increasing the elimination of toxic wastes through the skin. Saunas use dry heat to achieve this and can be used once or twice a week during detoxification. For most people, a sauna is a relaxing experience, quite apart from the desirable benefits of enhanced detoxification. A word of warning, though: coping with temperatures of 75-100°C involves a degree of physiological stress which should only be undertaken by the healthy.

An Epsom salt bath is also a highly efficacious sweat enhancer. Follow the instructions on p.67. Experiment with this and with packs and saunas to see which induces the greatest degree of perspiration while not leaving you tired – a fairly common effect of this form of detoxification, but which passes after a good night's sleep.

The full body pack, also known as the "Spanish mantle", is a slightly more elaborate version of the trunk pack described on p.67. It has two great advantages: the discolouration left on the sheet used is real evidence of the truly remarkable power of the method. And, once you have been wrapped in your body pack, you can go off to sleep – something you should not do in a sauna or bath.

Body pack
Take a single cotton sheet; wring it out in cold water, leaving it just damp. Spread it out on an open blanket and lie on it. Get someone to fold both materials over you thoroughly and firmly, so that you are parcelled up from the neck down. Have two or three hot water bottles placed inside the blanket, one near the feet, another about waist level and one higher up. Within ten minutes you should start to sweat profusely; within half an hour you will probably be asleep.

Three hours is the minimum for a full body pack. By then the sheet will be practically dry due to the hot water bottles and your insulated body heat. The sheet will contain strong acid wastes, so wash it thoroughly before re-use.

CAUTION: if you still feel cold after ten minutes, it will either be because the sheet was too wet or the insulating blanket not firmly enough wrapped around you. Get yourself released and try again another day.

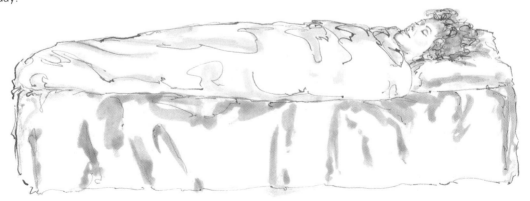

Face sauna

As you start to detoxify, and your body uses the skin as a route for elimination of wastes, blemishes or spots will probably develop on your face. A face sauna, or other home-made variations (see below), will greatly help detoxification and also encourage thorough cleansing of the pores.

One of water's remarkable properties is that each gram changed to steam retains 540 calories of stored heat. This heat is released when the steam condenses back into water. So, when you place your face over a sauna, the warmth of the condensation against your skin opens the pores and releases quantities of impurities and toxic waste through perspiration. The only equipment required is a kettle of boiling water, a bowl and a towel.

A drop or two of herbal extracts (below) in the bowl to which boiling water is being added, will ensure the presence of their essential oils in the steam. A less concentrated form of the herb would be obtained by boiling a few grams of the dried material in the water.

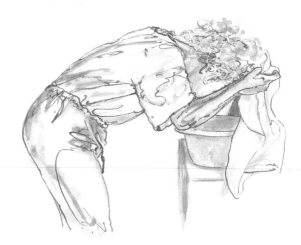

Pour boiling water into a bowl and cover your head with a towel to trap the steam. Stay under the towel up to ten minutes for maximum benefit, keeping the kettle handy to top up the water from time to time if it stops steaming. Afterwards, wash the face well with an alkaline soap (see p.127) and dab on a little diluted cider vinegar.

Variations with herbs and oils
Herbal extracts of linden blossom, rosemary or wild camomile are all excellent detoxifying agents. Add some to the water used in your face sauna. Mint, bay laurel and rosemary help tone the facial skin once impurities have been cleared.

Green clay
Fine French green clay (*argile sur fine*), obtainable at specialist health stores, is probably the best for attracting impurities. A paste of it spread on the facial skin whilst damp, dries hard and can be washed off some hours later, taking with it a vast amount of toxic waste.

How often?
First, try each of these methods to discover which you like best. Then use one – or alternate them – several times a week to keep the facial skin clear during active detoxification.

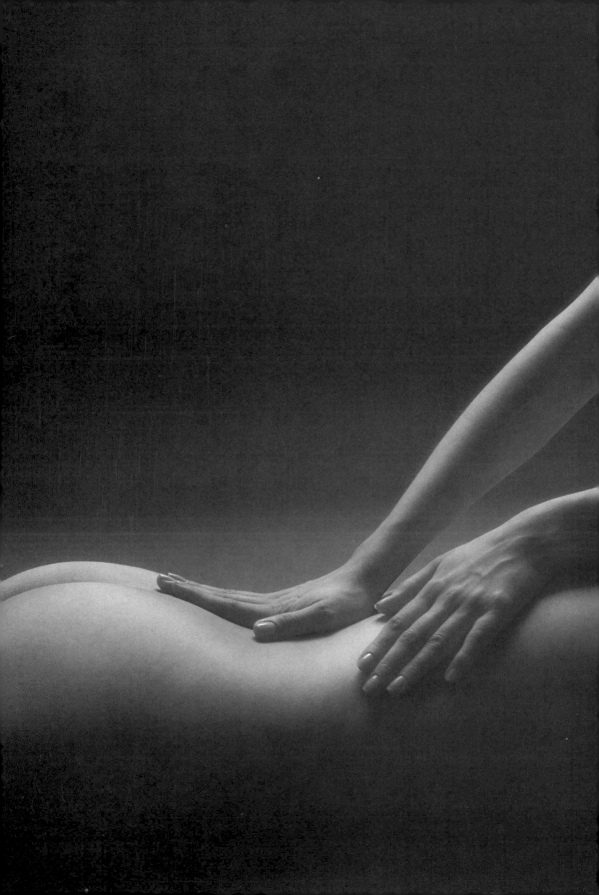

Massage

Massage is a marvellous technique for the release of tensions and the mechanical improvement of aspects of circulation, including lymphatic drainage.

Of all methods of treatment, few have the potential for safely removing tensions as massage. In order to achieve a relaxing effect, however, the massage strokes need to be purposeful and gentle and, above all, be given by someone who has both the intent and the patience to achieve that result. Unhurried, caring and thoughtful moves will usually produce relaxation. You will notice both a physical and an emotional element in the release of tensions when good massage is applied, and these are very closely linked. Muscles relax, circulation is improved, drainage is increased, tensions melt, and through all of these changes, detoxification is actively encouraged and helped.

There is usually a great depth of communication between the hands of the giver and the body of the receiver in sensitive body work, and this makes the intent of the giver profoundly important. There needs to be a desire to help, to soothe, to ease. Such nurturing emotions come best from someone who cares, ideally from a close friend or loved one.

Few experiences can match the emotional linkage which can take place between giver and receiver in massage, when this is performed in anything more than a mechanical way. Almost the most important aspect of massage is related to the intention of the giver. This sets the whole tone and pace of the massage. An "energy" interchange seems to take place which is dependent on the desire to nurture, support, care for and help the receiver, and this is transmitted through the medium of the hands of the giver.

Relaxation massage is especially useful in the early stages of a detoxification programme, doubly so if you are passing through the symptoms of withdrawal from habitually used substances, such as caffeine, tobacco, or alcohol. There is really no limit to how often such massage can usefully be employed.

The lymphatic drainage methods, which are also described in this chapter, involve a series of extremely slow, short, usually gentle, strokes. These are applied in order to help the movement of lymphatic fluid as it drains toxic wastes through the labyrinth of channels under the skin. Both surface and deep lymph drainage is useful, requiring variations in the amount of pressure used. Too much pressure overwhelms the capacity of the more superficial channels to handle the drainage effect. This kind of massage is most useful during the early detoxification stages, for reasons relating more to improving drainage than to relieving tensions.

Another form of massage uses specific pressure methods which are useful in helping to switch off painful trigger points which may be present. If an area of discomfort or pain is not more painful when you actually press it, then the pain sensations are probably being referred to that place from somewhere else. The painful region is called the target area and the source of the pain the trigger point. Treatment and self-treatment of such problems is very easy if you follow the guidelines given on the next page. Remember, massage should not produce pain; sometimes a "nice hurt", but never, in any circumstances, pain.

The principles of massage

Relaxation Massage   The simple effleurage (stroking) and wringing techniques on p.71-2 form the basis of relaxation massage. When using effleurage, try to get into a slow rhythmic pattern in which sometimes both hands go in the same direction and sometimes one hand moves across or down an area while the other is brought the other way. By slowly, rhythmically applying moderate pressure to muscles in this way, repeating strokes a number of times, circling the hands, gliding, stroking, lifting and wringing, a good deal of release can usually be felt of the tensions held by the muscles.

Similar patterns of massage can be applied to the legs, abdomen, chest and arms (see following pages). When working on the arms or legs, try to work from the extremity, towards the heart, thus moving the fluids in the same direction as the returning circulation.

After stroking and wringing is over, apply a light "feathering" series of strokes in which the fingertips lightly caress the skin. This has an almost incredible power to calm and relax the receiver.

Lymphatic Drainage   Wherever there is local fluid congestion, a very light (few ounces) stroking pressure with hand or thumb towards the heart, in a series of very slow (about seven a minute) movements, each travelling about two or three inches, will effectively reduce surface lymphatic accumulations after a few minutes.

When deeper lymphatic fluid needs moving, a heavier (few pounds) pressure applied in a series of equally slow moves towards the centre of the muscle, will help. Another useful lymphatic "pump" method is to combine deep slow breathing and clenching (on inhalation) of the fists and unclenching (on exhalation).

Trigger Points   As you massage yourself or your partner you may find small, lentil-sized, sensitive contractions which, on pressure, send painful sensations to areas some distance away. How to deal with these trigger points is described on p.181.

Apart from the pain symptoms they can cause, trigger points can also disrupt normal function in the target area to which they refer. This can lead to changes in skin texture, increasing any tendency for it to be dry or oily, or result in the sweat glands in the target area over-functioning, making the skin moist or clammy.

Trigger points
Dr Janet Travell, an American doctor who has researched trigger points for nearly fifty years, has discovered that many women suffering hot-flashes have this symptom abolished or much lessened when trigger points in their neck/shoulder area are effectively treated.

CAUTION: never apply direct pressure to the breast area, or to a lump or swelling.

Apart from lymphatic drainage, avoid having a massage during a fever.

Massage techniques

Massage can be either stimulating or relaxing. The effect will depend upon the degree of pressure and effort you use, and how slow and soothing, or vigorous and quick, the strokes are. Deciding which to apply depends largely on whether you aim to stimulate circulation, relieve stiffness or induce relaxation.

You have many strokes at your disposal. You can stroke muscles along their length; lift and wring them; deeply drain and stretch them, using the heel of your hand; vigorously run your fingers or thumbs across the fibres, lift and vibrate them, soothe and ease them...Strokes can be short and repetitive, long, circling or lengthening, quick or slow. You can use your whole hand, the heel of the hand, fingers or thumb to achieve the effect you wish. You can work on the skin surface itself, the muscles or deep into the underlying fascia. And you can ring the changes from one variation to another, relying on your intuition, sensing what is needed. Remember, though, that you should never hurt your partner – except in trigger point work where a slight degree of discomfort is inevitable.

When you give a massage, use a suitable oil or lotion to avoid skin-drag. Numerous oils are now available containing essential oils such as those used in aromatherapy. These greatly enhance relaxation or other effects. Too much will cause you to slither and slide and be unable to control the hand contacts; too little irritates the skin, pulls the hair, and prevents rhythmic movement of the hands.

Kneading and wringing:
Use your whole hand to grasp, slightly lift and squeeze bunches of muscle tissue. This calls for one hand to release its grip as the next takes over on another segment of the muscle. Develop a rhythmic, rocking sequence, as the hands alternate their activity, just as in bread making.

Use the same hand position for wringing: both hands grasp tissue simultaneously and put the tissue between the hands gently into slight torsion, like wringing out a towel.

As an alternative, pull one hand towards you as the other pushes away, stretching the muscle between the hands. Make these moves slowly, never hurting.

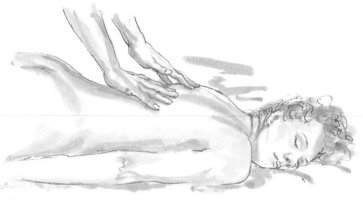

Feathering:
After any massage work, apply a series of fingertip contacts in which you "feather" down the area worked on. With hands totally relaxed, alternately brush the tips lightly over the skin, drawing your hands towards you, one after the other. As one long stroke finishes, the next begins, barely touching the skin. This needs to be a very slow movement, repeated as many times as you wish until, ideally, you see your partner's breathing calm to a slow, shallow level, or there is a deep, releasing sigh.

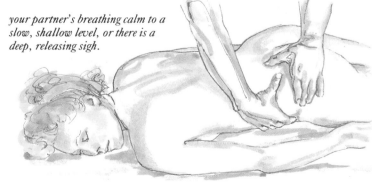

Relaxation massage

Apart from someone to give and receive it, you will need a warm, quiet room, a suitable surface on which to lie, no distracting noises, and, above all, no time constraints. Allow enough time for a slow return to normal after the massage, so that the relaxation it produces can be savoured and enjoyed. Sleep may well follow.

If the person being massaged is to lie face down, try to have a cushion under the abdomen to prevent the low back sagging, and a small pad under the ankles. If face up, have the knees lightly bent or supported by a cushion.

The person giving the massage must make sure that the strokes are thoughtful, slow, rhythmical and fluid, so that one movement leads into the next. Avoid jerky, mechanical movements.

Always keep at least one hand on your partner once you begin. As you work through the different regions of the body, some will feel more tense than others. Spend more time here, feeling for the signs of release or relaxation, and using intuition to guide you as to when you have done enough, and it is time to move to another area. Have the intention of presenting your partner with an experience which comes from your caring touch.

This sequence describes massage of both the back and front of the body. It is not essential to massage both at the same session unless you want to and have the time.

If you have dealt with the feet, for example, in the back sequence, it is obviously not necessary to work on them again during front massage.

Take great care not to put pressure on the breasts and apply only easily tolerable amounts of pressure to the abdomen.

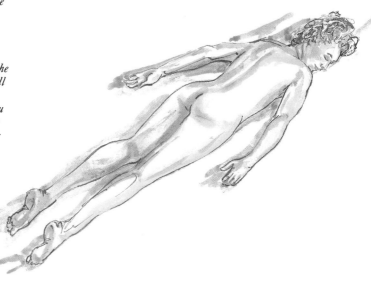

Lie your partner face down. Take some minutes to apply a warm lotion or oil to the area you will first be working on. Kneel at the head, and with a series of firm, long, unhurried, strokes, apply the lubricant to the skin of the neck all the way down to the small of the back (which is about as far as you can comfortably reach from your position at the head). Relax your hands, and mould them to the contours of the tissues they touch.

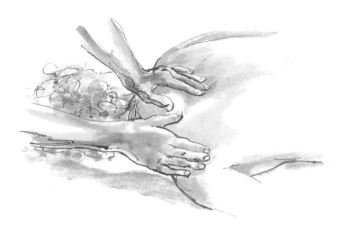

First strokes

Let both hands travel down the back, one on each side of the spine, to about the middle of the back, where they separate to curve down to the sides of the ribs, before coming up again to the start at the base of the neck. The next stroke should be further out from the spine, but following a similar route. These contacts, mainly with the whole palm or heel of the hand, have a general firm stroking quality, feeling for differences in tension and smoothing them out.

Kneading the shoulder

Use your hands alternately to lift and knead the tissues between the shoulder and the neck. This is an extremely sensitive region, so use a minimum of force. In some places you will be able to get hold of tissue with the whole hand, whereas in others only between finger and thumb can you lift and squeeze the muscles. Travel round and over the shoulder blade, doing this to all tense tissues.

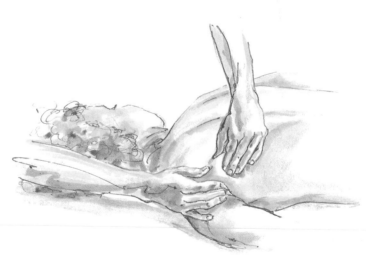

Searching deeper

After the initial general stroking and wringing/stretching, start to search deeper with your thumb for tense and tight regions in the muscles under the surface. The most important area in the upper body is around the base of the neck, and towards the shoulder blade. Also apply this searching, releasing pressure from the spine outwards, all the way from the base of the neck to the middle back. If you find "trigger points" which refer pain elsewhere (this is a major hunting ground for them), see p.170.

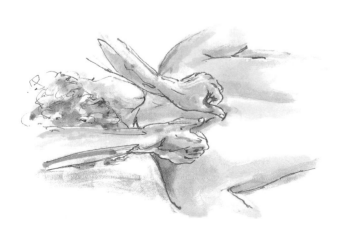

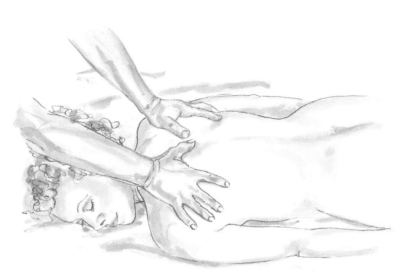

Outwards from the spine

After deep thumb searching, repeat some of the original general strokes to calm and soothe the region massaged so far. Apply a series of strokes using the whole hand, moulded to the body contours, which take the hands down the spine and out over the lower ribs before returning to the starting position. Then apply strokes outwards from the spine, over the shoulder blades followed by a series running from the spine towards the hips. Use the heel of the hand gently to come across the muscles which lie alongside the spine, stretching them carefully away from it.

Wringing low back muscles

Now move to the side, so that you can lean over and across your partner, using both hands to apply a series of wringing, lifting, stretching holds and strokes to the muscles of the low back. The large buttock muscles should also receive attention from this position. Deep rhythmic work is a powerful aid to release of tensions locked into this important part of the body.

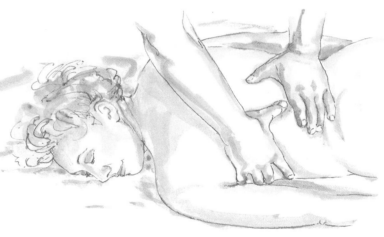

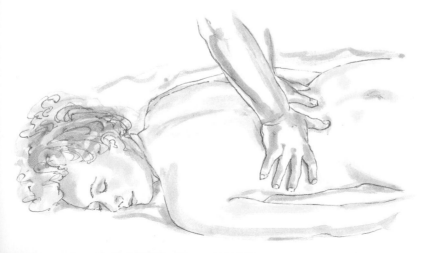

Moving to the waist

Leaning further over your partner, use a similar series of whole-hand strokes to stretch the muscles of the lower back, applying pressure both downwards parallel with the spine and also outwards across the large muscle groups and down to the sides. As you get to the limit of your reach, you should be able to give some heel of hand attention to the upper buttock region, where a great deal of sensitivity is often found.

Thighs

Kneel at the level of your partner's knees, facing slightly towards the head. Apply oil or lotion to the (bent and supported) leg and use an alternating series of lifting, squeezing, wringing moves to release tension in these muscles. Mould your hands to the contours, and try to establish a slow, rhythmic pattern as you work from the knee towards the hip. Pay attention to the muscles at the side of the upper leg, as tension here is common. Finish with a series of long strokes which "milk" the tissues upwards from knee to buttock.

Lower leg

Starting just above the ankle, lift and wring the muscles of the calf as you rhythmically travel towards the knee. Keeping an even pressure, go up and down these muscles several times, avoiding any pressure on varicose veins. Finish with a series of whole-hand strokes, draining the muscles upwards towards the knee.

Foot

Supporting it with one hand while you work with the other, take your time to search the sole of the foot with sensitive thumb pressure. Exquisitely sensitive areas can be found here, and it is often ticklish. You therefore need to make a slow, strong but not painful contact. Work around the ankle and between the bones which you will feel in the toe region. The most important part is under the arch, where you can produce a lot of relief by diligent thumb and finger work.

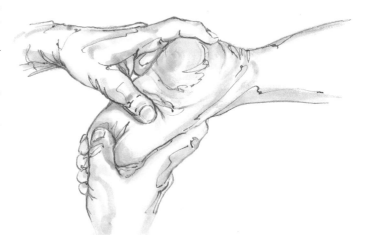

Face

Keep a steady, uniform degree of light pressure throughout your massaging of the face. This requires sensitivity. Use thumbs to massage from the centre of the forehead outwards from the eyebrows to the hairline, and above. Lightly massage from the eyebrows over the eyes and stroke the thumbs out over the cheekbones, continue outwards from the nose, the upper lip, mouth and chin. Circle and ease the muscles of the jaw. Finish with heel of hand contacts over the cheekbones, forehead and down onto the neck. Ease the muscles there by lifting and stretching.

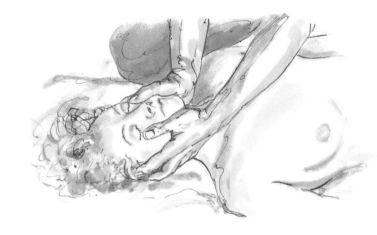

Shoulders

Use both hands to work on the muscles of the shoulder, including those leading into it from the front and behind. These tissues are sensitive, and contacts with the heel of the hand and whole palm are less likely to irritate than are the thumbs. Place one hand under and one over the shoulder and lift and stretch it gently, circling it while you knead the muscles.

Arm

Cradling the arm, use long, slow strokes, with your hand moulded to the arm contours, to drain the muscles towards the shoulder. Lift, wring, knead and stretch the muscles between the hand and shoulder, both along the length of the arm and across the fibres where-ever tension is most obvious (usually the forearms). Work on the hand as you did on the foot, with most emphasis on the palm, and using your thumbs to stretch the muscles which work the fingers.

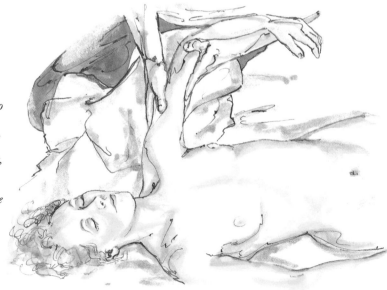

Chest

These muscles are vital to normal breathing function and deserve special attention. From the head, lean over your partner and use either heel of hand contact to stretch the muscles outwards from the centre, or finger contacts to lift and stretch from the sides upwards towards the centre. Avoid direct pressure on the breasts when working on a female partner. Lift and gently knead the muscles which run up into the shoulder from the breast bone, but remember how sensitive they are. To finish, perform a series of slow, circular or long hand contact strokes to soothe and calm the muscles you have worked on.

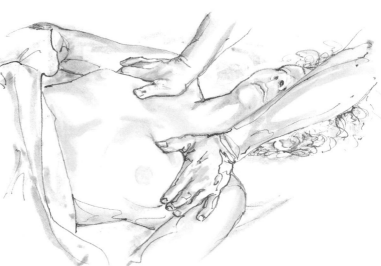

Abdomen

Kneeling one side, use both hands to circle the abdomen so that as one hand comes towards you, the other moves away. One hand stays in constant contact as it circles clockwise, while the other is lifted off as the hands cross. Work slowly and progressively deeper with the heel or palm of the hand. The pressure used will depend upon the sensitivity of your partner. Much emotional tension is locked into these muscles; sighing and changes of breathing rhythm are a sign of its release.

Diaphragm

Apply gentle but steady pressure upwards on the diaphragm with the fingers or heel of hand as your partner breathes deeply and slowly. Increase the pressure slightly each time he/she breathes out, maintaining pressure on the inhalation. Do this for around ten full cycles of breathing (in and out) to help relax this vital area. Slight discomfort (but not pain) is usual.

Thighs

Position yourself to the side, or between the legs of, your partner, so that the leg being worked on can be easily approached and lubricated. Use both hands alternately to stroke upwards from the knee to the hip region, draining the tissues. Use the whole hand as well as the thumbs to circle, wring and stretch the muscles from the centre of the leg to the sides. After working with the thumbs around the knee-cap, and with the whole hand on the important muscles around the hip joint, finish with long, slow contacts which stretch the thighs.

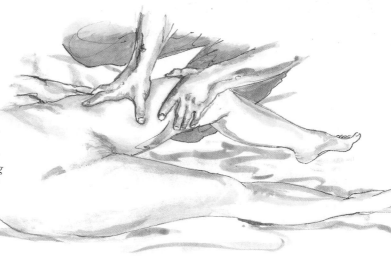

Shins

The muscles alongside the shinbones are very sensitive. As you apply a series of deliberate, rhythmical strokes upwards from the foot towards the knee, and also across these muscles, outwards from the centre, with the thumb or heel of hand, be careful to use no more pressure than is easily tolerable to your partner. Support the knee with a cushion to relax the lower leg muscles. Finish with a soothing series of strokes, always upwards.

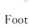

Foot

The final contact of a massage is usually with the feet. With fingers under the sole, and heel of hand on the front of the foot, apply a rhythmical squeezing as you separate your hands to stretch the small bones gently apart. Work with the thumbs around the ankle and then apply gentle stretching to the toes. Finish by holding the heel firmly with one hand as you stroke upwards over the front of the foot.

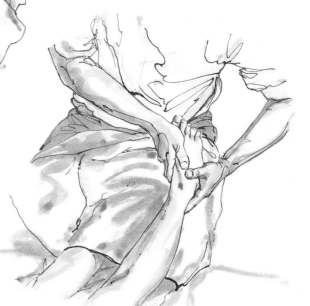

Lymphatic circulation

Lymph is the clear fluid which circulates through the channels of the lymphatic system, acting as a carrier of wastes. These wastes are filtered out of the lymph at the lymph nodes, special sites arranged in long strings and clusters. The detoxified lymph which passes through the chains of nodes is later gathered together as it passes through special drainage ducts.

As pressure builds up in the lymph channels, a wave-like muscular contraction (peristalsis, like the movement which moves the contents of the digestive tract) moves it along. If pressure is too high, for example as a result of the sort of congestion of the lymph glands you feel in your throat when you have flu or a cold, there is an overload of the drainage potential, and a degree of stagnation occurs. This can be

The 600-plus lymph nodes in the body (over 150 in the neck region alone) are both filtering stations and manufacturing sites for important protective cells, the lymphocytes, which protect against invading organisms. The nodes ensure that lymph is purified of toxins and invading organisms before it passes through the major drainage ducts on its way back into the blood system.

The lymph channels are the drainage system of the body, independent of, and yet linked with, blood circulation.

Lymph flows through tiny channels which link up with larger drainage conduits, finally reaching lymph nodes. Here the lymph is cleansed, and antibodies produced to neutralise any foreign invaders carried in the lymph. After cleansing, the lymph passes again into the bloodstream through ducts in the upper body.

The more toxic you are, and the less exercise you have, the greater the stagnation of the lymphatic circulation, which depends greatly on mechanical pumping by muscle and breathing activity to keep it moving. Anything you do to improve breathing and movement will improve drainage. Stretching, breathing and aerobic exercise will help, as will massage. For the deeper lymph structures, this means directing massage strokes from the ends towards the centre of a muscle. For surface drainage, try to massage towards the nearest large nodes (illustrated).

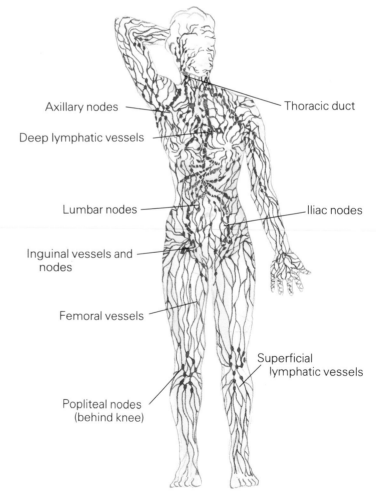

Axillary nodes

Deep lymphatic vessels

Lumbar nodes

Inguinal vessels and nodes

Femoral vessels

Popliteal nodes (behind knee)

Thoracic duct

Iliac nodes

Superficial lymphatic vessels

helped by slow, gentle massage, ideally in the direction of flow of the lymph. If the massage is too vigorous or heavy, it will overload the system, so go slow, go light (see p.170).

The direction of the arrows shows you the way lymph travels as it clears the body of wastes and foreign sub-stances (toxins and bacteria). Slow, stroking massage (see p.170) in these directions will assist the drainage function, as does deep breathing and exercise.

Front   Back

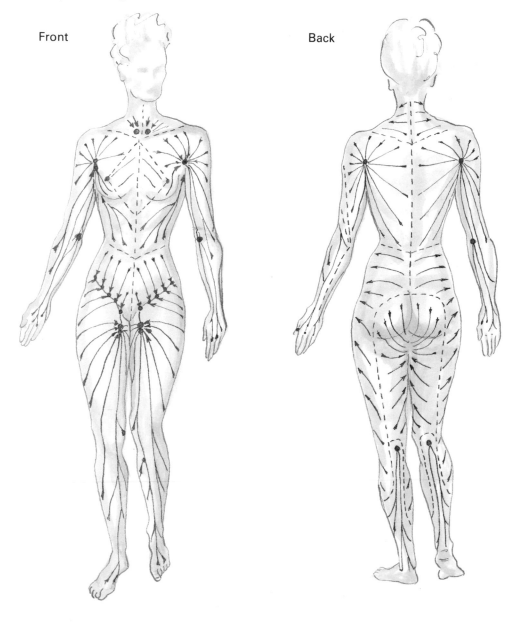

Trigger points

Sensitive areas in muscles resulting from local stress or injury can become the source of pain and problems in distant tissues. These local areas are called trigger points. If you find sensitive areas during massage, and if, when pressed, they radiate pain or discomfort to a target area some distance away, apply just enough pressure to the point to produce the referred symptoms. After a minute's pressure, or so, gently stretch the muscle in which the trigger point lies.

In some areas, such as the neck, you should not apply direct pressure. Rather, squeeze the point to produce the referred symptoms. The importance of these areas in detoxification is that, until they are resolved, the area cannot relax And if it cannot relax physically, you cannot relax mentally. And detox calls for body and mind to release and relax.

Note: not all sensitive points will radiate in this way – only active trigger points.

Pressing
Find a local area of sensitivity and press with finger or thumb tip until a distant area registers pain. Hold pressure for a minute and then stretch the muscle in which the trigger is found.

Pinching
Take a muscle region (neck, shoulder) in which a local area of sensitivity has been found; grasp the tissue between finger and thumb and squeeze until (a) local discomfort is felt, and (b) a distant (head or hand) sensation is felt. Hold for a minute and then stretch the muscle in which the trigger lies.

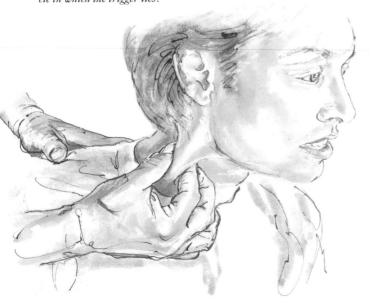

CAUTION: never apply pressure on a lump or swelling, on the breast, on a varicose vein, or where the skin is broken. Never apply enough pressure to cause more than background referred pain, and never press hard enough to bruise.

Cleansing the system

Enema An enema removes toxic wastes from the lower bowel. This is specially important during a fast, whether or not you have had a normal movement. You can use either a syringe (from any pharmacy) or a gravity bag to get water into the lower bowel.

Syringe: Lie on your right side, with your knees bent, on a thick towel. Lubricate the end of the applicator with a sterile jelly and slowly ease the end of the tube past the anus into the rectum. Slowly squeeze the syringe containing water at body heat and, over a period of several minutes, take in about a quart. Take it slowly; it can produce a cramping sensation if hurried. Massage the abdomen gently if you have any feelings of gas pressure. Turn onto your left side for a few minutes as well. Try to retain the water for at least five minutes before voiding it into the toilet.

Gravity bag: Hang this, containing about a quart of warm water, about two feet above the level at which you are lying. Insert the end of the applicator tube as described above, lying on your right side. Release the clamp on the tube, allowing water to flow gently into the rectum. If there is any discomfort, clamp it off and massage the abdomen for a moment. When the discomfort passes, resume the flow until a quart has been absorbed. After five minutes or so void the water into the toilet.

Coffee enema This unusual use of coffee is not to clear the lower bowel, but to stimulate your liver to rid itself of toxin-laden bile. Take three tablespoonsful of ground (not instant) coffee and add a quart of water. Boil it for three minutes and allow it to stand for another fifteen. Use a quarter of this (half a pint) at body heat as an enema (above) as often as you feel the need to relieve nausea and general feelings of tiredness and lethargy.

Acidophilus enema If Candida is a problem (p.38), dissolve a large teaspoonful of high-potency acidophilus powder in a quart of water and use it in an enema as described above. Retain for fifteen minutes, if possible, before voiding. This type of enema is not meant to clear the bowel, but to help repopulate the lower bowel with "friendly" bacteria which destroy invasive yeast such as Candida.

Coping with cravings

Many of the unhealthy habits we commonly use – eating sweet or starchy foods, smoking, drinking and drugging – rely on the sugar/adrenalin cycle for their attraction. Breaking into this pattern is therefore desirable, and there are quite a few steps you can take to help.

● **Sugar**

A craving for sweet things is likely to be related to low blood sugar problems and/or stress and stimulant-related adrenal gland exhaustion (see p. 18).

Two grams of the amino acid L-glutamine has been shown to reduce sugar (and alcohol) craving in nine out of ten people. Take it in divided doses (away from meal times, with water).

If sugar-craving is also associated with a highly stressed state and exhaustion, take 1-2 grams of vitamin C daily with meals and a high potency supplement of vitamin B complex, with a meal.

In addition, to assist adrenal gland recovery, the B vitamin, Pantothenic acid, should be taken individually (in the commonly available form of calcium pantothenate) at a dose of 500 milligrams, to be taken with food at a separate time from the B complex.

Animal and human studies have shown that one gram of the amino acid tryptophan (take it on a piece of bread about 20 minutes before a meal) can reduce the desire for starchy/sweet foods and increase the desire for savoury/protein foods at that meal. (Tryptophan is turned into serotonin and transported to the brain where it influences food choice.)

If low blood sugar is apparent, take 500 microgrammes daily of the mineral chromium (richly supplied in liver, brewers yeast, black pepper and wheatgerm).

● **Caffeine**

Caffeine is present in tea, cola drinks, cocoa and chocolate, as well as coffee. Reliance on these stimulants often involves an unconscious attempt to increase sugar levels in the blood and production of adrenalin for a boost in energy. The result is, all too often, hypoglycaemia and adrenal exhaustion. Follow the advice given for sugar, while caffeine intake is being cut back or eliminated.

● Nicotine

Nicotine also has the effect of stimulating sugar release (via adrenalin) into the bloodstream, and, since most tobacco is sugar-cured, it also causes sugar present in the smoke to reach the bloodstream almost as soon as it is inhaled. The same hypoglycaemic connection can be applied to tobacco usage as to caffeine (and alcohol) dependence.

There is often a direct ritual connection between smoking and habits of coffee or tea drinking, and also to the intake of highly spiced foods. For several week after stopping smoking (and ideally for a week or so before) stop consuming all stimulant beverages and highly seasoned foods.

Supplements which assist in the recovery of the body from smoking and which also ease withdrawal symptoms include:

Vitamin A – 15,000 iu daily
Vitamin C – not less than 2 grams daily
Vitamin E – 400 iu daily
Vitamin B3 (niacinamide) – 500 milligrams daily
Vitamin B5 (calcium pantothenate) – 500 mg daily

High potency B-complex (containing not less than 50mg each of major B vitamins such as thiamine and riboflavin) – one daily taken at a meal and away from either B3 or B5, which should also be taken separately from each other.

Acupuncture or acupressure is recommended to help ease withdrawal problems of any sort.

● Tranquilizers

It is not commonly realized that one of the major effects of taking tranquilizers. is the rapid release of sugar into the bloodstream. Coming off tranquilizers is not easy, and should not be undertaken without medical advice or the assistance of a support group or counsellor. However, the nutritional advice given for dealing with sugar will be helpful. Follow a high protein/high complex carbohydrate diet; as in all low blood sugar related problems eating little and often is better than large meals widely spaced.

Resources

ENVIRONMENT

Barnaby, Frank *The Gaia Peace Atlas* (Pan Books, UK, 1988; Doubleday, US, 1988)

Bates, W H *Better Eyesight without Glasses* (Grafton, UK, 1979; H Holt, US, 1988)

Bunyard, Peter, *Health Guide for the Nuclear Age* (Macmillan, UK, 1988)

Button, J., *Green Pages* (MacDonald Optima, UK, 1988), *The Green Guide to England* (Green Print, UK, 1989) and *How to be Green* (Century, UK, 1989)

Chaitow, Leon *The Radiation Protection Plan* (Thorsons, UK, 1989)

Christensen, Karen *Home Ecology* (Arlington Books, UK, 1989)

Concern Inc (ed) *Drinking Water – A Community Action Guide* (Washington DC, 1986)

Cook, Judith *Dirty Water* (Unwin Hyman, UK, 1989)

Curwell, S R and Marsh, C G (eds) *Hazardous Building Materials, A Guide to the Selection of Alternatives* (E & F N Spon, UK, 1986)

Dadd, Debra Lynn *Non-toxic & Natural* (J P Tarcher, US, 1984) and *The Nontoxic Home* (J P Tarcher, US, 1986)

Davidson, John H., *Radiation: What It Is, How It Affects Us And What We Can Do About It* (C W Daniel, UK, 1986)

Dudley, Nigel *The Poisoned Earth* (Piatkus, UK, 1987)

Durrell, Lee *State of the Ark* (Bodley Head, UK, 1986; Doubleday, US, 1986)

Elkington, John, Burke, Tom, and Hailes, Julia *Green Pages* (MacDonald Optima, UK, 1988)

Elkington, John and Hailes, Julia *The Green Consumer Guide* (Gollancz, London, UK, 1988) and *The Green Consumer's Supermarket Shopping Guide* (Gollancz, 1989)

Friends of the Earth *A-Z of Local Pollution* (London, 1988) and *The Good Wood Guide* (London, 1988)

Golos, Natalie and Goblitz, Frances *Coping with Your Allergies* (Simon & Schuster, US, 1986) *The Householder's Guide to Radon* (HMSO, London, June 1988)

Huxley, Anthony *Green Inheritance* (Collins, UK, 1984; Doubleday, US, 1984)

Lambert, Barrie *How Safe is Safe?* (Unwin Hyman, UK, 1990)

McConville, Brigid *The Parents' Green Guide* (Pandora Press, UK, 1990)

Mendelsohn, Robert *How to Raise a Healthy Child in Spite of Your Doctor* (Contemporary Books, US, 1984)

Mumby, Keith *Allergies: What Everyone Should Know* (Unwin Hyman, UK, 1986)

Myers, Norman (gen ed) *The Gaia Atlas of Planet Management* (Pan Books, UK, 1985; Doubleday, US, 1984)

Ott, John *Health and Light* (Pocket Books, US, 1982) and *Light, Radiation and You* (Devin-Adair, US, 1985)

Pearson, David *The Natural House Book* (Conran Octopus, UK, 1989; Simon & Schuster, US, 1989; A. & R. Collins, Aus)

Porritt, Jonathan (ed) *Friends of the Earth Handbook* (MacDonald Optima, UK, 1987), *Seeing Green* (Blackwell, UK, 1984), and *The Coming of the Greens* (Collins, UK, 1988)

Rousseau, David, Rea, W J, and Enwright, Jean *Your Home, Your Health, and Well-Being* (Ten Speed Press, US, 1988) (available from Airlift Book Co *see* below)

Samuels, Mike and Bennett, Hal Zina *Well Body, Well Earth* (Sierra Club Books, US, 1983)

Venolia, Carol *Healing Environments* (Celestial Arts, US, 1988) (available in UK from Airlift Book Co *see* below)

Webb, Tony *Radiation and Your Health* (Camden Press, UK, 1988)

Worldwatch Institute, Brown, Lester R et al. *State of the World* (W W Norton, US, 1988)

HEALTH

Bahr, Frank *Acupressure: A Complete Guide to Health and Pain Control* (Unwin Hyman, UK, 1982)

Bates, W H *Better Eyesight without Glasses* (Grafton, UK, 1979; H Holt, US, 1988)

Davis, Adelle *Let's Get Well* (Unwin Hyman, UK, 1974) and *Let's Stay Healthy* (Unwin Hyman, UK, 1983)

Homeopathic Development Fund, *Homeopathy: The Family Handbook* (Unwin Hyman, UK, 1987)

Hunter, Myra *Your Menopause* (Pandora Press, UK, 1990)

Kenton, Leslie, *Ultrahealth* (Ebury Press, UK, 1984), *The Joy of Beauty* (Century, UK, 1983), and *Ageless Ageing* (Century, 1985)

Mabey, Richard *The Complete New Herbal* (Elm Tree, UK, 1988) and as *The New Age Herbalist* (Collier Books, US, 1988)

McCormick, Elizabeth *The Heart Attack Recovery Book* (Unwin Hyman, UK, 1987)

O'Sullivan, Sue *Women's Health: A Spare Rib Reader* (Pandora Press, UK, 1987)

Priest, Judy *Drugs in Pregnancy and Childbirth* (Pandora Press, UK, 1990)

Richardson, Diane *Safer Sex* (Pandora Press, UK, 1990)

Scott, Julian *Natural Medicine for Children* (Unwin Hyman, UK, 1990; Avon Books, US, 1990)

Stanway, Dr Andrew (gen ed) *The Natural Family Doctor* (Century, UK, 1987; Simon & Schuster, US, 1987)

Winterson, Jeanette *Fit for the Future* (Pandora Press, UK, 1986)

DIET

Budd, Martin *Low Blood Sugar* (Thorsons, UK, 1987)

Campbell, Susan, *The Cook's Companion* Mac-Millan, UK, 1980)

Cannon, Geoffrey and Lawrence, Felicity *Additives: Your Complete Survival Guide* (Century, UK, 1986)

Canter, D, Canter, K, and Swan, S *The Cranks Recipe Book* (J M Dent, UK, 1982)

Chaitow, Leon *Amino Acids in Therapy* (Thorsons, UK, 1985), *Candida Albicans: Could Yeast Be Your Problem* (Thorsons, 1985), and *Stone Age Diet* (Optima MacDonald, UK, 1987)

Davis, Adelle *Let's Cook It Right* (Unwin Hyman, UK, 1979) and *Let's Eat Right to Keep Fit* (1974)

Drew, Smith and Mabey, David *The Good Food Directory* (Hodder & Stoughton, UK, 1986)

Ewald, Ellen, *Recipes for a Small Planet* (Ballantine, US, 1973) (available in UK from Wholefood, 24 Paddington Street, London W1)

Gear, Alan *The New Organic Food Guide* (Dent, UK, 1987)

Hanssen, Maurice *The New E for Additives* (Thorsons, UK, 1987)

Grant, D and Joice J *Food Combining for Health* (Thorsons, UK, 1984)

Grigson, J., *Vegetable Book* (Michael Joseph, UK, 1978) and *Fruit Book* (Michael Joseph, UK, 1982)

Hunt, Janet *The Holistic Cook* (Thorsons, UK, 1986)

Katzen, Mollie *The Moosewood Cookbook* (Ten Speed Press, US, 1977) and *The Enchanted Broccoli Forest* (Ten Speed Press, 1982) (available in the UK from Airlift Book Co *see* below)

Kinderlehrer, J., *Confessions of a Sneaky Organic Cook...or How to Make Your Family Healthy while they're not looking* (Rodale, US, 1971)

Lobstein, Tim, The London Food's Commission *Children's Food* (Unwin Hyman, UK, 1988)

Look Again at the Label (available from The Soil Association Ltd., 86-8 Colston Street, Bristol BS1 5BB)

London Food Commission *Food Adulteration and How to Beat it* (Unwin Hyman, UK, 1988)

Maisner, Paulette with Turner, Rosemary *The Food Trap: A Self Help Plan to Control Your Eating Habits* (Unwin Hyman, UK, 1986)

Moore Lappe, Frances *Diet for a Small Planet* (Ballantine, US, 1982) (available from Wholefood, 24 Paddington Street, London W1)

Mott, Lawrie and Snyder, Karen *Pesticide Alert* (Sierra Club Books, US, 1987)

Mumby, Keith *The Food Allergy Plan* (Unwin Hyman, UK, 1985)

Myers, Judy, *Staying Sober* (Simon & Schuster, US, 1987)

Smith, Drew and David Mabey (eds) *The Good Food Directory* (Consumers' Association, London, UK, 1987)

Snell, Peter *Pesticide Residues in Food* (London Food Commission, 1986)

Spencer, Colin *The New Vegetarian* (Elm Tree Books, UK, ; Viking, US)

Stanway, Dr Penny *Diet for Common Ailments* (Sidgwick & Jackson, UK, 1989) and as *Foods for Common Ailments* (Simon & Schuster, US, 1989)

Thomas, Anna *The Vegetarian Epicure* (Penguin, UK, 1973)

Webb, Tony and Lang, Dr Tim, *Food Irradiation: The Facts* (Thorsons, UK, 1987)

MIND DETOXIFICATION

Books

Alcoholics Anonymous (Acoholics Anonymous, 1939, annually updated)

Black, Claudia, *It Will Never Happen to Me* (M.A.C., US, 1981)

Chaitow, Leon *Your Complete Stress Proofing Programme* (Thorsons, UK, 1985)

Crabtree, Tom *Tom Crabtree's Guide to Coping* (Unwin Hyman, UK, 1987)

Dyer, Wayne W., *Your Erroneous Zones* (Funk & Wagnalls, US, 1976)

Kirsta, Alix, *The Book of Stress Survival* (Unwin Hyman, UK, 1986; Simon & Schuster, US,

1986) Lake, T and Acheson, F *Room to Listen, Room to Talk: A Guide to Analysis, Therapy, and Counselling* (Bedford Square Press, UK, 1988)

Mason, L John *Guide to Stress Reduction* (Celestial Arts, US, 1985) (available in the UK from Airlift Book Co *see* below)

McCormick, Elizabeth *Nervous Breakdown* (Unwin Hyman, UK, 1988)

Melville, Joy *First Aid in Mental Health* (Unwin Hyman, UK, 1984)

Milam, James R. with Ketcham, Katherine *Under the Influence* (Bantam, US, 1983)

Postle, Denis, *The Mind Gymnasium* (Macmillan, UK, 1988; MacGraw Hill, US, 1988; A & R Collins, Aus, 1988)

Reid, Howard *The Way of Harmony* (Unwin Hyman, UK, 1988)

Roet, Brian *Hypnosis: a Gateway to Better Health* (J.M. Dent, UK, 1986), *All in the Mind? Think Yourself Better* (Macdonald Optima, UK, 1987), *A Safer Place to Cry* (1989)

Waxman, David *Hypnosis* (Unwin Hyman, UK, 1984)

Whitfield, Charles, *Healing the Child Within* (Health Communications, US 1987)

Wilde McCormick, Elizabeth *Change for the Better* (Unwin Hyman, UK, 1990)

Wilson, Mary *Living With a Drinker* (Pandora Press, UK, 1989)

Wholey, Dennis, *The Courage to Change* (Houghton Mifflin, US, 1984)

Winston, Stephanie *Getting Organized* (Warner, US, 1978)

Organizations

Alcoholics Anonymous, General Service Office, PO Box 1, Stonebow House, Stonebow, York YO1 2NJ, UK. Tel: 0904 644026. London Region Telephone Service, 11 Redcliffe Gardens, London, SW10. Tel: (01) 352 3001

Alcoholics Anonymous, General Service Office, 468 Park Avenue South, New York, NY 10016, USA. Tel: (212) 686 1100

Al-Anon Family Groups, 61 Great Dover Street, London, SE1, UK. Tel: (01) 403 0888

Al-Anon Group Headquarters, PO Box 182, Madison Square Station, New York, NY 10010, USA. Tel: (212) 302 7240

British Association for Counselling, 37A Sheep Street, Rugby CV21 3BX. Tel: 0788 78328 (for directory of counselling and psychotherapy organizations)

Narcotics Anonymous, PO Box 417, London

SW10 0RS, UK. Tel: (01) 351 6794

Narcotics Anonymous, PO Box 622, Sun Valley, CA 93352, USA. Tel: (818) 780 3951

Tranx (UK) Ltd. National Tranquilizer Advice Centre. Tel: 01 427 2827 (24 hour answering service) and 25a Masons Avenue, Wealdstone, Harrow, Mix. 01 427 2065

EXERCISE, BREATHING, WATER THERAPIES, & MASSAGE

Balaskas, J *Natural Pregnancy* (Sidgwick & Jackson, UK, 1990; Interlink, US, 1990; Simon & Schuster, Aus, 1990)

Ewald, Hans, *Acupressure Technique for Self-Treatment of Minor Ailments* (Thorsons, UK 1978)

Lidell, Lucy *The Book Of Massage* (Ebury Press, UK, 1984; Simon & Schuster, US, 1984) and *The Sensual Body* (Unwin Hyman, UK, 1987; Simon & Schuster, US, 1987)

Myers, Judy, *Staying Sober* (Simon & Schuster, US, 1987)

Reid, Howard *The Way Of Harmony* (Unwin Hyman, UK, 1988); Simon & Schuster, US, 1988)

Sivananda Yoga Centre *The Book of Yoga* (Ebury Press, UK, 1983) and as *The Sivananda Companion to Yoga* (Simon & Schuster, US, 1983)

Thomas, Sara *Massage for Common Ailments* (Sidgwick & Jackson, UK, 1989; Simon & Schuster, US, 1989; A. & R. Collins, Aus, 1989)

Tisserand, Robert *The Art of Aromatherapy* (C W Daniel, UK, 1977) and *Aromatherapy for Everyone* (Penguin, UK, 1988)

MAIL-ORDER BOOK SUPPLIERS

For UK:

Books for a Change, 52 Charing Cross Road, London WC2H OBB. Tel: (01) 836 2315

Schumacher Book Service, Food House, Hartland, Bideford, Devon EX39 6EE. Tel: (02374) 293

Airlift Book Co., 26 Eden Grove, London N7 8EF. Tel: (01) 607 5792 (UK distributors for US publishers: North Point, Celestial Arts, and Ten Speed Press Books)

For US and UK:

Whole Earth Access (WEA), 2990 Seventh Street, Berkeley, CA 94710, USA.

Index

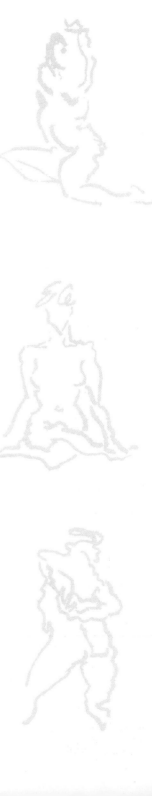

Photographic credits
Robyn Beeche pp.13, 21, 30, 93, 96, 148. Fausto Dorelli pp.7, 11, 15, 42, 55, 130, 168. Camera Press p.59. Images Colour Library pp.16, 25, 115, 119, 158. Ted Polhemus p.112. Tony Stone World-wide pp.3, 135, 165.

Acknowledgements
Gaia would like to thank Norman Myers and Sara Martin for their help and advice. Sarah Menon for design, Ann Chasseaud for illustration, Robyn Beeche and Fausto Dorelli (and their models Peter Davey, Karen Drumy, Peter Warren, Polly Eltes, and Trish Nolan) for photography. The team – Lynette Beckford, Penny Cowdrey, Jonathan Hilton, Rosanne Hooper, Libby Hoseason, Sara Mathews, Terry Moynaighan, Samantha Nunn, Joss Pearson, Susan Walby, Eve Webster – and especially Gian Douglas Home for Resources, Leslie Gilbert for copy preparation, Michele Staple for the index, and On Yer Bike.

Typesetting: Cambridge Photosetting Services

Colour reproduction: Fotographics